This is a story many of us have eagerly awaited, and there is no one better suited to tell it than Damian McElrath and John Curtiss. They eloquently depict the conditions that spawned the idea of The Retreat, how that idea grew into a community, and how that community has evolved. This is a story with profound implications for the future of addiction treatment and its viability and status as a cultural institution. That alone makes this book noteworthy, but of even greater importance are the profound implications this story has on the future of addiction recovery in the United States and beyond.

The wake of this book will bring animated discussion and debate about what distinguishes a recovery community from a treatment program, mutual help from professional help, communities of recovery from healthcare organizations, and the comparative merits of sophistication versus simplicity. No one should enter that conversation without first reading this book.

—**William L. White**, author: *Slaying the Dragon: The History of Addiction Treatment and Recovery in America*

The founding of The Retreat is one of the most significant events in the treatment of addiction in the last thirty years. This book reveals the spiritual heart of the The Retreat and the countless lives it's saved. A treasure.

—**Jeff Jay**, coauthor of *Love First: A Family's Guide to Intervention* and author of *At Wit's End: What You Need to Know When a Loved One Is Diagnosed with Addiction and Mental Illness*

This compelling story of The Retreat, told by Damian McElrath and John Curtiss, should give us all hope that recovery from alcohol and drug dependency can be affordable, accessible and effective for all who need it. This time-tested "caring community" approach to recovery has become a standard of care that has helped thousands of individuals and their families access a life of recovery. This book provides an historical perspective of the Minnesota Model of treatment, the impact of managed care on the treatment field and chronicles the step-by-step process this group of dedicated addiction professionals and recovered individuals undertook to change the way people access a life of meaningful and productive recovery.

—**Christopher Kennedy Lawford**, author:
What Addicts Know; Recover to Live; Symptoms of Withdrawal; and *Moments of Clarity.*

As our nation continues to struggle to find more afford-able and effective strategies to help the millions of individuals and families who suffer from alcoholism and drug dependency The Retreat has become one of the most promising solutions on the addiction care land-scape. I have been honored to have been with both Dr. George Mann and John Curtiss from the beginning as they dreamed about what The Retreat could become and ultimately made the dream a reality. The world needs to pay close attention to this model of care. The Retreat is one of the most promising solutions we have seen in decades to addressing our nation's number-one health-related problem.

—**Jim Ramstad**, former congressman and co chair of the Addiction, Treatment and Recovery Caucus

There has been no story in the addiction treatment field in the past decade that has been more compelling or presented a greater opportunity to save more lives than The Retreat's "caring community" approach. With dignity and respect, The Retreat allows those with a desire to recover from their alcoholism and drug dependency to connect to a vibrant community of men and women who are living recovery at the highest levels. This model has proven to be the magic formula for making recovery effective, affordable and accessible. That experience helps provide the spiritual growth necessary to recover.

I'm grateful to consider myself part of The Retreat's caring Community.

—**Andrew Zimmern**, author, teacher, chef and creator of Travel Channel's *Bizarre Foods with Andrew Zimmern*

This isn't simply the story of The Retreat. This book brings us back to the truth of recovery. In reading these pages, I repeatedly stopped to give silent thanks to John Curtiss and Damian McElrath for writing them. It's as if they are outstretching their hands to the reader and saying, "Here is the treasure we were given. It is for us to protect it, preserve it, and share it." It comes from their deep understanding that treatment must serve the recovery communities of Alcoholics Anonymous, not the other way around.

—**Debra Jay,** author of *No More Letting Go: The Spirituality of Taking Action Against Alcoholism and Drug Addiction,* coauthor of *Love First: A Family's Guide to Intervention.*

a caring community
the story of the retreat

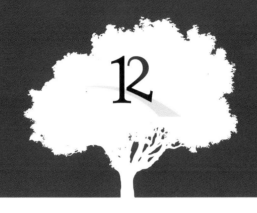

A REVOLUTION
IN THE TREATMENT
OF ALCOHOLISM AND
DRUG DEPENDENCY

DAMIAN McELRATH
& JOHN CURTISS

foreword by William L. White

BEAVER'S
POND
PRESS

ISBN 13: 978-1-59298-920-1

Library of Congress Catalog Number: 2014910783

Printed in the United States of America

First Printing: 2014

18   17   16   15   14   5   4   3   2   1

Cover design by Judd Einan, Fluence Creative
Interior design by James Monroe Design, LLC.

BEAVER'S
POND
PRESS

Beaver's Pond Press, Inc.
7108 Ohms Lane
Edina, MN 55439–2129
(952) 829-8818
www.BeaversPondPress.com

To order, visit www.BeaversPondBooks.com
or call (800) 901-3480. Reseller discounts available.

Anonymity is a blessed tradition in the AA community. We've consulted with many people in pulling the threads of this story together. We thank them all. The flaws in this book are ours—not theirs.

Dedicated to our friend and guiding light, Dr. George Mann, without whose steadfast commitment and leadership The Retreat might never have happened.

And to the hundreds of AA and Al-Anon volunteers who give of their time and their hearts to carry the message of hope and recovery to all we serve.

Contents

Foreword

We must begin to create naturally occurring, healing environments that provide some of the corrective experiences that are vital for recovery.

—SANDRA BLOOM, CREATING SANCTUARY

There is a pervasive theme in the more than 280-year history of addiction treatment and recovery in the United States: when structures of recovery support collapse or get diverted from their recovery mission, recovering people, their family members, and a vanguard of professional allies will rise to forge new structures of recovery support. That theme is vividly illustrated in the history of The Retreat.

The founding of Alcoholics Anonymous (AA) in 1935 brought new hope for a condition that had long been plagued with pessimism. The pre-AA world was one in which alcoholics were more likely to receive contempt than care from the professional community. In the 1940s, recovering people and their allies, under the leadership of Mrs. Marty Mann, launched a movement to change the way America viewed alcoholism and the alcoholic. More than three decades of sustained advocacy led to federal legislation in 1970 that laid the foundation for modern addiction treatment. That emerging treatment system included widespread replication of the Minnesota model of chemical dependency treatment—a model that drew heavily from AA's unique program of alcoholism recovery.

The founding vision of the 1940s recovery advocacy movement was of an ever-growing recovery community. Movement leaders viewed professional treatment as an adjunctive linkage—a portal of entry for the sickest of the sick—into a community of mutual support.

Hundreds of thousands of lives were subsequently touched and transformed by the emerging treatment system, but within twenty years of its rise, the advocates who were the godparents of that system were questioning what their life's work had wrought. What they saw was a multibillion-dollar treatment industry that viewed recovery as an afterthought and adjunct to itself—if at all. It is not possible to understand The Retreat without understanding the soil in which it grew.

Voices began to rise in the 1990s suggesting that addiction treatment had become disconnected from the larger and more enduring process of addiction recovery as well as from the grassroots communities out of which it was born. Long-tenured addiction counselors began to fear that something very important had been lost on the road to the professionalization and commercialization of addiction treatment. The signs of such loss were evident in many quarters. Recovery representation declined among addiction counselors, and the legions of recovering volunteers disappeared amidst the new wave of professionalism. Relationships eroded between addiction treatment organizations and AA and other recovery mutual aid fellowships. Addiction became viewed not as a primary disorder but a superficial manifestation of underlying psychopathology. The emphasis on spirituality and the power of a caring community declined in tandem with growing interests in dual diagnosis, an ever-expanding service menu, and the use of psychotropic and anticraving medications. The language of the heart was displaced by a new vocabulary that tenured counselors castigated as "psychobabble."

The ultimate loyalty of many treatment organizations shifted from those being served to those regulating and paying for service. Concern for recovery rates gave way in many organizations to concerns about census rates and profit margins. In this new climate, counselors lamented spending more time on paperwork than people work. Treatment became ever briefer, and long-term recovery became less and less of a visible focus of addiction treatment. In response to these changes in the field's essential character, spiritual leaders within the addiction treatment field suggested it was time to conduct a searching and fearless moral inventory and that perhaps the field was itself in need of a recovery process.

Such sentiments contributed to the rise of a new recovery advocacy movement in the late 1990s that, as it developed, challenged the treatment field to renew its recovery orientation. Simultaneously, experiments were initiated to recapture the best within the founding visions of addiction treatment, particularly from within the earliest era of the Minnesota model. In that process, approaches to recovery support were created (or re-created) that defined themselves not as professionally directed addiction treatment but as spiritually focused communities of mutual recovery support. Among the earliest proponents of this approach were Dr. George Mann and John Curtiss, whose shared vision took life in 1998 in The Retreat. Mann and Curtiss drew on their mutual concern over the direction of addiction treatment and their long, respective tenures at St. Mary's Hospital and Hazelden to recapture the purity and simplicity of what they felt had been lost in the evolution of the Minnesota model and the larger arena of modern addiction treatment. Their vision was of an approach focused exclusively on addiction recovery that was spiritually based, affordable, accessible, and effective. The boldness of what The Retreat created was not in forging a new form of treatment; it was in building a community of mutual help that no longer defined itself as treatment. It was in creating a community in which a contagious spirit of recovery rose not from the direction of a professional but from this caring community.

The subsequent success of The Retreat has prompted numerous efforts, nationally and internationally, at replication and adaptation, but the story of the history and inner workings of The Retreat has, until now, not been told. Nor has there been any detailed presentation of how The Retreat was influenced by, and yet differs from, Hazelden and other exemplars of the Minnesota model. This is a story many of us have eagerly awaited, and there is no one better suited to tell it than Damian McElrath and John Curtiss. In the following pages, they eloquently depict the conditions that spawned the idea of The Retreat, how that idea grew into a community, and how that community has evolved. This is a story with profound implications for the future of addiction treatment and its viability and status as a cultural institution. That alone makes this book noteworthy, but of even greater importance are the profound implications this story has on the future of addiction recovery in the United States and beyond.

The wake of this book will bring animated discussion and debate about what distinguishes a recovery community from a treatment program, mutual help from professional help, communities of recovery from health-care organizations, and the comparative merits of sophistication versus simplicity. No one should enter that conversation without first reading this book.

—William L. White
Author, *Slaying the Dragon:*
The History of Addiction Treatment
and Recovery in America

Preface

When the Community of Recovering People (CORP) was founded in 1991, the professional treatment field was in serious decline. But there was no decline in the number of people needing help and the negative effect these numbers had on the social, economic, and spiritual dimensions of American society.

The task confronting the founding members of the Community of Recovering People was a formidable one. CORP evolved because millions of people were not getting the help they needed due to the internal and external barriers that had evolved over the previous two decades. External pressures were squeezing the life out of the treatment field. Treatment was simply too costly, making it inaccessible for most. Other internal factors were moving treatment in directions that not only were inordinately expensive but also appeared to challenge the simple model of treating a primary disease—alcoholism or chemical dependency. Many millions could not get help that was affordable, accessible, and effective—the three key objectives that evolved to become the spiritually based mission of The Retreat.

For the first four years, the members of CORP struggled with how they would accomplish these three objectives. It took the men and women who made up CORP some seven years to discover and bring about their model of mutual help. The journey took seven years of dead ends, wrong turns, and unchartered roads. It was to be a recovery program, but not a professional treatment program. What evolved was a radically different approach to helping the alcohol-and drug-dependent person and their families. The inspiration and perseverance for the journey derived from the crucible of their own personal recoveries, particularly in imitation of the mutual help that Bill W. and Dr. Bob provided for one another. This, in the final analysis, became the model for The Retreat. With the writing of the twelve traditions, Bill W. made it clear that his movement was not to be institutionalized but was to remain a spiritual community, a fellowship of mutual help. In contrast with the other treatment programs that had preceded it, The Retreat represents the model of a caring community, a "we" program, a community that centers on the mutual help of like-minded people.

In the 1970s and 1980s, the Minnesota model was acknowledged to be the preeminent model of treatment. It provided an invaluable service to the care of chemically dependent people in the United States. But much of its luster has diminished as it has sought to recapture its preeminence by multiplying its services to treat the whole person. By so doing, with expanded professional staffing, it drifted from the simple mutual help program as it was conceived in 1948–49, modeled by both Pat Cronin at Pioneer House and Lynn Carroll at Hazelden. (See epilogue.)

But the expansion of this treatment model eventually stopped and went into rapid decline, not because it ceased being effective, but due to a confluence of external forces. State licensure and national accreditation requirements weighed heavily upon treatment centers, which wanted only to deliver a simple message of recovery. The medical and psychological components of the Minnesota model played increasingly more important and time-consuming roles in the treatment of patients who were presenting with more co-occurring disorders, a development commonly referred to as "Complexity." The multiplication of services and the increase in basic and supplemental fees raised the cost of treatment beyond what many could pay unless they had insurance. Insurance, for its part, with the help of managed-care companies, sought to exercise cost control with a host of admission requirements, the most challenging of which were subjective interpretations of medical necessity and preexisting conditions.

In one sense, The Retreat is a re-creation of the

Minnesota model in its pristine form. In that sense, it represents the earliest stages of a model that recapture much of early AA, with its reliance on the AA community and its investigation of the richness of *Alcoholics Anonymous: The Big Book* and the Kit of Spiritual Tools—the Twelve Steps. This healing protocol of a caring community and the Twelve Steps bring to the fore the simple truth that recovery is all about the rediscovery of the relationships with our real selves, with others, and with the God of our understanding.

Dr. Bob's walk in recovery began in his relationship with another drunk (*Alcoholics Anonymous*, 180), not with a book or a workshop on alcoholism. His conversation with Bill W. set the stage both for an individual's recovery and for a recovery movement. The core of recovery rests on the premise of what truly makes us human—to be in relationship with others. In this case, their fellowship carried the day over the next four years. During that time, Bill W. gave form to that principle of relationship in composing *Alcoholics Anonymous: The Big Book*. In it, he encapsulated the mutual help principle in a Higher Power, the Twelve Steps, and the powerful stories of recovery to drive home the principle of powerlessness and the solution that was to be found in others. The framework for delivering the message of recovery was in mutual help settings—meetings in the Wilson home in New York, the Williams's home, St. Thomas Hospital in Akron, and the Club at 2218 in Minneapolis. This tradition initiated by Bill W. and Dr. Bob has become richly endowed over the decades in similar meetings throughout the world.

In a final essay, this book will trace the evolution of the recovery model in Minnesota from its great pioneer, Pat Cronin, and his model of mutual help at 2218 to professional treatment as encompassed by the Minnesota model. It will be clearly seen that this caring community model found in The Retreat, geographically located in Minnesota, seeks a return to the basics of mutual help, one alcoholic helping another, as discovered by Bill W. and Dr. Bob.

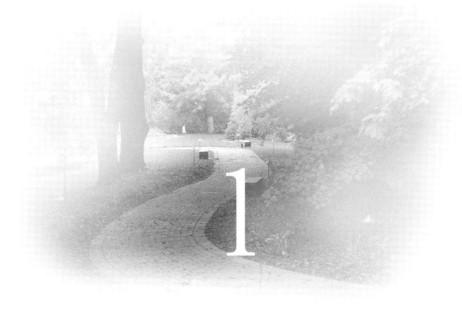

Chaos in the Treatment Field

In June 1991, a group of dedicated men and women calling themselves the Community of Recovery came together to review the purpose of their meeting. They found that they were basically in agreement about a crisis in the treatment field and about their desire to do something. There was a need to return to basics in helping chemically dependent people and making this help available to people at a sustainable cost. The group was formally incorporated the following February under the official title "The Community of Recovering People." Its mission was very straightforward: "CORP is dedicated to the development of services that will assist people as they begin sobriety and will enhance the lives of people already in sobriety."

In that same year, 1992, the cost and consequences of alcoholism and drug dependence placed an enormous burden on the United States. As the nation's number-one health problem, addiction strained the health-care system and the economy, harmed family life, and threatened public safety. Substance abuse crossed all societal boundaries—both genders, all ethnic groups, and every tax bracket. Then, scientific documentation defined alcoholism and drug dependence as a disease with roots in both genetic susceptibility and personal behavior.

In terms of actual numbers, the economic cost to society from alcohol and drug abuse in 1992 was an estimated $246 billion, of which alcoholism and alcohol abuse cost $148 billion, while drug dependence and abuse cost an estimated $98 billion in lost productivity, health-care expenditures, crime, motor vehicle crashes, and other conditions. (From 1985 to 1992, the economic costs of alcoholism and alcohol abuse alone had risen 42 percent.) About 18 million Americans had alcohol problems, and about 5 million had drug problems.

In 1992, more than 132,000 people died as a consequence of alcoholic and drug problems—107,400 from alcohol abuse and 25,500 from drug abuse. Much of the economic burden of alcohol and drug problems fell primarily on the population that did not abuse alcohol and drugs. Every American that year paid nearly a thousand dollars for the damages of addiction.

Scientific evidence demonstrated that treatment for

alcohol and drug abuse worked. It not only saved lives, but also saved dollars that would otherwise be spent in other areas of medical and social services. For every dollar spent on addiction treatment in 1992, $7 was saved in reduced health-care costs. (In 2013, the savings were estimated to be $16 for every dollar spent on treatment.) But the fact of the matter was that only a small percentage of the population was receiving treatment at the time that CORP was founded.

Not only were the numbers small, but also the treatment industry for chemical dependency was in serious crisis. William White in his monumental work, *Slaying the Dragon: The History of Addiction Treatment and Recovery in America*, describes the treatment field as being in panic, in chaos, and in search of its soul. Occupancy rates for private inpatient programs were in steep decline between 1989 and 1993; hospitals either merged their psychiatric and addiction treatment units or exchanged their inpatient units for less costly outpatient programs; successful treatment was not always measured by outcomes but by occupancy rates (White, 284–87).

During the 1990s, there was a period of reassessment. From one viewpoint, that was exactly what CORP was engaged in from 1991 until 1998, when it opened the doors of The Retreat. Initially, CORP did not have a clear vision of what path to follow in helping the chemically dependent—the challenges and needs appeared insurmountable.

The specific problems that CORP was reacting to are easily discernible in the lives of two of its members, although all of the directors had similar backgrounds. In the early years of treatment in Minnesota, John Curtiss, president of The Retreat, and George Mann, the inspiration for and chairman of CORP, experienced chemical dependency treatment as simple and uncomplicated. Both of them had worked for preeminent centers of treatment, Curtiss as vice president of Hazelden's National Continuum, and Mann as the director in charge of chemical dependency services at St. Mary's Hospital.

Looking back, all of the directors realized how unencumbered treatment had been without the regulatory demands and the chokehold of managed care. Things were simple. Individuals and families got well, and their gratitude was enduring. But then things changed and the simplicity of the treatment field was lost in a maze of rules and regulations, the mandates laid down by managed care, and the multiplication of services within the treatment setting—services that came under the umbrella of "treating the whole person." It took a while for CORP to disengage from the model that had been in place in Minnesota for close to four decades. This was the Minnesota model of treatment, a model of national and international fame. That disengagement occurred at the very time the Minnesota model was being seriously challenged.

Insurance companies had never been pleased with Minnesota's early 1970s mandate that all insurance premiums carry a minimum of twenty-eight days of residential treatment for chemical dependency. What particularly disturbed them was that the growing number of treatment centers were completely unregulated when Minnesota passed the insurance requirement.

There were no accepted criteria for diagnosing alcoholism and chemical dependency nor was there a set of standards to determine which institutions and counselors were professionally qualified to treat alcoholics. It was not long, however, before the response to these concerns was the creation of national accreditation programs, state licensing standards, and the development of counselor training and credentialing.

But just when it seemed that the treatment of chemical dependency was gaining respect and confidence, insurance companies expressed further concern at the bills that were being charged to them. At first they simply sought discounts in the contracts they negotiated with treatment centers. The next stage created the most pain. They hired companies to manage the reimbursement provided for care. And with implementation of managed care, the vast network of treatment that had been built up over two decades slowly began to crumble.

What happened? Managed care, quite simply, was the delivery of health care in an environment where both utilization and price could be directly influenced and managed by companies hired for that purpose. The consolidation, health surveillance, and concentration of control and power that managed care was soon to exercise had a serious effect on the treatment field. In Minnesota, Blue Cross/Blue Shield began to move aggressively to rein in health-care costs, particularly in the areas of mental health and chemical dependency.

By the mid-1980s, the insurance companies had managed to bypass mandated coverage by insisting that patients demonstrate medical necessity. The criteria for medical necessity were determined by the managed-care company, which often made them so stringent and narrow that only a small percentage of patients seeking treatment could qualify. Medical necessity, together with the denial of coverage for preexisting conditions, permitted insurance companies, through managed care, to erect formidable barriers to the case for treatment.

To satisfy insurance requirements, treatment centers added adjunct staff at considerable cost and developed standards for admission, continued stay, and discharge under the headings of Utilization Review, Quality Assurance, and Total Quality Management. All became top priorities for treatment centers. The insurance companies, and their managed-care agents, countered this by usurping the program's Utilization Review and other programs as untrustworthy and assumed for themselves a precertification function to verify medical necessity and rule out preexisting conditions for which insurance could not be used. Treatment programs were forced to retreat further and further.

The gate-keeping practices of managed care inevitably took its toll. Occupancy rates for private treatment centers (insurance supported) and hospitals plummeted between 1991 and 1993. Residential programs with solid traditions and alumni bases relied on private pay clients (a fee out of reach for many) and contracts with managed-care companies at reduced admission fees.

As Damian McElrath (1999, 51) wrote: "The insurance industry, chafing under the rash of reduced profits, shed its diapers and donned the boxer shorts of managed care to begin cuffing the ears of the mental and chemical health fields, looking for an opportunity for delivering a knockout blow. The treatment field began to feel the effects of this pummeling and centers began to close at an accelerating rate in the late eighties and early nineties." Health-care initiatives under the Clinton administration kept the doors ajar, but with their failure, the future of the treatment industry looked gloomy indeed. It was the survival of the fittest or those with a strong alumni base such as Hazelden, Caron, and Betty Ford Center.

Some traditional professionals in the treatment field lent their own voices to the protestations against treatment, proclaiming that it was ineffective; that abstinence was unrealistic, inhuman, even un-American; and that the disease concept of alcoholism was the figment of someone's fertile imagination. In the mid-1970s, the Rand Report had trumpeted research about the value of controlled drinking. Now, in the late 1980s, the banner of the efficacy of controlled drinking was unfurled once again to the satisfaction of those who felt that loss of control was a myth because there wasn't anything that Americans could not do if they set their minds and their wills to it.

The media joined in and highlighted the abuses, especially regarding the treatment of adolescents, shunting to the side decades of dedicated service. Adolescent/young adult treatment at St. Mary's and Hazelden Pioneer House, along with other programs throughout Minnesota, underwent serious scrutiny by the national media and government agencies in the late 1980s. The charge directed against these treatment centers—in a few cases proven, but in most cases not—was that they were improperly diagnosing and admitting young people, especially those from other states, into residential treatment and holding them there to keep their beds full.

The insurance industry did have some legitimate grievances against the treatment providers. In the early 1980s, hospital administrators were desperate to fill their beds and the insurance-covered chemical-dependency industry seemed especially lucrative. At the same time, treatment centers and clinics proliferated and there was fierce competition to maintain a high census and fill beds. Marketing practices could be creative but often misleading in their promises. Addictions multiplied and anyone rumored to be addicted was a likely candidate for treatment. Some referrals were misdiagnosed, over diagnosed, or not diagnosed at all.

It should be noted that the growth of the treatment field before the existence of CORP was staggering, increasing from a handful of programs in the 1950s to 2,400 programs in 1977, almost 7,000 in 1987, and 9,057 in 1991 (White, 276). As more and more for-profit organizations entered the field, in some cases quarterly dividends rather than treatment outcomes were the major concern. When inpatient programs ceased to make a profit and revenues continued to shrink, hospitals turned to outpatient programs for the chemically dependent. St. Mary's, where Dr. George Mann had served for two decades in charge of its chemical dependency programs, was one of these.

The Alcoholics Anonymous (AA) community, which many treatment centers were seeking to assist in the recovery process, had some very negative observations. Filling beds, treatment in general, and the money motive did not sit well with AA. Not only had the recovery model moved from mutual help to professional treatment, but for-profit organizations were making money on the alcoholics' problems.

Many felt treatment centers were corrupting AA and accused them of employing therapeutic buzzwords and "psychobabble," the language that their graduates were using in place of the solid AA slogans at meetings. Instead of the healthy AA laughter used to poke fun at oneself (and others), graduates from treatment programs were full of "angst" and continually whining about their "injured selves." The old timers referred to the mountains of commercialized literature as "recovery porn" (White, 278).

Some of the problems for the treatment field arose with the increase of a multidisciplinary staff (an essential feature of the Minnesota model), in response to what was believed to be the multidimensional nature of the disease of chemical dependency. Besides the medical nature of detoxification, which naturally required the presence of doctors and nurses, soon it was decided that the patients would need the services of psychologists to determine whether or not mental health was an issue.

In the early stages of the evolution of the Minnesota model, if the answer was yes, the problem was relegated to an aftercare (continuing) care plan, unless the problem was so severe that it demanded an immediate outside referral. Initially, the role of the psychologist was to interpret the Minnesota Multiphasic Personality Inventory and identify concerns or personality traits that needed watching so as not to interfere with an individual's ability to participate in treatment.

In the 1980s, the *Diagnostic and Statistical Manual of Mental Disorders*, third edition, created the framework for the development of services for individuals with co-occurring disorders. In 1987 the National Institute for Mental Health recommended that co-occurring disorders be treated concurrently. One of the recommended models of such an approach to treatment was an "integrated" formula that would address both the chemical dependency and the mental health concurrently within the same system. This was the path some treatment settings took to respond to the challenge of acuity. The most common of the mental health issues were mood and anxiety disorders, e.g., major depression, posttraumatic stress, and social phobia. John Curtiss and others felt the introduction of the dual disorder framework, however vital and important for some, tended to over-pathologize the disease of chemical dependency and might eventually relegate it to the rank of a secondary disorder.

The United States is a drug-seeking society, with a pharmaceutical industry only too ready and willing to satisfy that appetite. The patients are more knowledgeable and more sophisticated when it comes to medications and pharmacology. It is not unusual for patients to come to treatment on any number of medications unrelated to illegal mood altering chemicals.

Integrating co-occurring disorders into the treatment plan provided a serious challenge to the simplicity of the Minnesota model. Still more challenging is the reality that it is the brain's reward system that drives one to use alcohol or other chemicals in larger and more frequent doses to get increased stimuli. Many mental health professionals came to believe that to treat addiction with only fellowship or psychotherapy is to address the fight on only one front. They believed that to deal adequately with the disease, the new model should have two parts: stabilization of the chemical system and focused counseling to teach the rest of the brain the necessary coping strategies for change. Without counseling, stabilization is only temporary. Both approaches need to go hand in hand. The challenge of medication therapies is twofold: poor adherence to the dosing protocols may result in a high relapse rate and the medication therapy alone will ignore the fellowship, psychotherapeutic, and spiritual components essential to the recovery process.

Brain research has been providing the field with a great deal of information that needed to be translated into treatment practice, i.e., using approved medications for patients experiencing intense craving, a biochemical, physiological response to alcohol and chemicals. These anticraving medications have documented some effectiveness, and there is hope for additional medications on the horizon. As they become available, general practice physicians who have little training or experience in addiction medicine would almost certainly prescribe them. While all of these medications are recommended as simply components of social/spiritual treatment, the reality and threat are that it will not always happen that way.

The Federal Drug Administration's approval of anticraving medications for alcohol dependence (acamprosate and naltrexone) opened up what could become the Pandora's box for treatment. Some professionals in the treatment field feel the drugs are another clear step toward the introduction of a medical model that further blurs the line between the medical and the Twelve Step approach to recovery. At the same time, the very preliminary data does show that particular pharmaceuticals prescribed for alcohol do help sustain the recovery process.

None of these medications are as effective if they are not accompanied by counseling or talk therapy. Ideally, anticraving medications are intended to reduce relapse and improve recovery rates by integrating medication use with treatment protocols. For some time, the medication model had been thought of as a threat to the Minnesota model of recovery. The jury is still out as to whether the medications will be used in conjunction with the Twelve Step program or will replace its inclusion in future treatment protocols. The worry is that anticraving medications are just another step toward transforming abstinence-based/Twelve Step treatment programs into medical models of treatment or even worse, eliminating them as an option all together.

It took a long time for alcoholism to be recognized

as a primary illness, not a secondary result of a mental health problem. In the early days of treatment, mental health problems that were detected in treatment were seen as either derivative from the alcohol diagnosis or continuing care problems. Then, as mental health problems persisted, the co-occurring paradigm took over, and those problems were given time in the treatment process, sometimes equal time. It remains to be seen if a future challenge will reemerge: a return to the belief that alcoholism is not a primary disease but secondary to the co-occurring mental disorder.

A more subtle internal problem had been the continuing education and growing expertise of the counselors, which quietly changed the dynamic between the patient and the clinician. There was a time in the early days of treatment or mutual help programs that the only credentials for assisting the patient were that the helper had a good recovery and could lecture/talk well about his/her experience, strength and hope. Some believe that initial relational/mutual quality emblematic of a caring community has been replaced by a more educated and sophisticated clinician characteristic of a treatment program. There are those who believe that something may have been lost in the evolution.

It is difficult to capture all the variables of the backdrop on which The Retreat is to be presented. It was an extraordinarily challenging time for the treatment industry.

It took time, but George Mann and John Curtiss gradually identified the barriers that their new solution would address. Cost was a major one. But initially it was their belief that a less clinical, more spiritual, heart-centered solution was needed. To their credit, the two solutions arrived together. By addressing and removing the cost-producing elements of the model in combination with mutual sharing, they had a new formula: returning to the older sharing model, using *Alcoholics Anonymous: The Big Book* as a core curriculum, making alcoholism and addiction primary versus a shared co-occurring focus of treatment, shifting from the clinical or medical focus to a spiritually based model of mutual sharing, staffing only with those whose individual recovery was primary, and adding a large volunteer base to carry this message. How this all came together is woven in the life experiences of the two main founders of The Retreat: George Mann and John Curtiss.

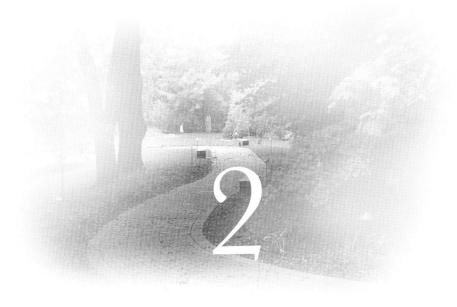

George Mann, MD,
St. Mary's Hospital

The story of The Retreat starts with Dr. George Mann, who played the preeminent role in its past and present evolution, which together give the spark and lay the foundation for its future. Before the initial soundings about a new model of recovery, Dr. Mann spent two decades fashioning a recovery program at St. Mary's Hospital in Minneapolis, Minnesota, which had the distinction of initiating one of the earliest and most prestigious hospital-based chemical dependency programs in the United States. It grew in knowledge and wisdom under his guidance as medical director. He brought together a team of competent individuals with a special concern for addicted persons. Together they developed a treatment program that provided high-quality services for chemically dependent people and their families. But the program was not born and nurtured without difficulty.

What is very telling and paradoxical about the hospital's excellent treatment program was that Mann in his early career as a physician knew hardly anything about alcoholism or chemical dependency. The manner in which he came to learn about dependency and its pernicious consequences was highly personal and painful.

Mann graduated from medical school at the University of Minnesota in 1947 with a specialty in anesthesiology. At that time, the subject of alcoholism found hardly a place in the curriculum. It was only a decade later, in 1957, that the American Medical Association decided to list alcoholism as a disease. Mann said that the general feeling among the doctors was that an assignment to the emergency room to detox the alcoholics was looked upon as a punishment. The "drunks" were a nuisance and needed to be shown the revolving doors of the hospital as quickly as possible. However, the time did come when St. Mary's created a model of care that respected the dignity of the alcoholics, similar to the care and respect that St. Thomas Hospital in Akron, Ohio, afforded under the guidance of Dr. Bob and Sister Ignatia. (See epilogue.)

During his early years at St. Mary's, Mann was regarded as a hardworking and very dependable doctor, highly esteemed by his fellow physicians. While raising a large and loving family, he recalled that something "awful" was happening to his lovely wife. In particular, he became aware of her drinking habit and the effects it was having on their family and especially her relationship with him. His wife's unabated drinking and the unmanageability that ensued covered a decade that he described as the worst of his life. It got so bad that eventually he dreaded going home at night. It came to the point that his wife's psychiatrist suggested that he get a divorce. But before he entertained anything so drastic, he began his own case study by observing her symptoms and trying to determine what might be the cause of them.

Staying up one night well into the morning hours poring over his medical books in conjunction with his wife's behavior, it finally dawned on him that his wife was an alcoholic. Having conferred with others about where to get help, in the latter part of 1966 he brought her to Hazelden, where she spent a month on the unit called Dia Linn, meaning "God be with you." (The women patients had been recently transferred from Dellwood, near White Bear Lake, to the Center City campus on Good Friday 1966. It was referred to as "Black Friday" by those who thought the decision was a poor one with ominous implications. They believed the clever placement of bear traps throughout the campus would not keep the men and women apart. As a result of the merger, the future looked bleak for Hazelden in the eyes of many.)

After his wife had been there for three or four days, she called her husband and said: "George, do you know what is wrong with me? I am sick." Then she repeated it once again. "I am sick. I have an illness." That was the beginning of her recovery journey, which continued with her participation in Vern Johnson's new after-care services. (Johnson had worked as a chaplain at Dia Linn, and later at Center City, hearing fifth steps and delivering lectures. He then embarked on his own career and eventually founded the Johnson Institute. His pioneering work with families influenced the direction the family program took at St. Mary's.)

When his wife returned home, the hopes of a loving family were rekindled. The interactions of the whole family grew progressively better and more loving as their journey continued to unfold before them. (Mann reminisced that the more than forty-five years of her continuing recovery were the happiest decades of his life.)

Dr. Mann continued to enjoy his work as an anesthesiologist at St. Mary's. In 1968, his life suddenly and radically changed. He attended a talk by Marty Mann, the first lady of Alcoholics Anonymous (AA) and the founder of the National Council on Alcoholism. Upon Marty's recovery, she dedicated her life to helping alcoholics and to spreading the word about AA and its vast potential for recovery. Her audience was a cross-section of the medical community in the Twin Cities. During the course of her presentation, she reminded those present that they were the people primarily responsible for the health care of their community. Yet there was a large segment of it not receiving care for a serious disease—chemical dependency. (By this time, addiction to alcohol and drugs came under the general heading of "chemical dependency.")

George Mann, whose gratitude for his wife's recovery was unlimited, was so impressed by the power of Marty Mann's words that the next day he walked into the office of the president of St. Mary's, Sister Mary Madonna Ashton, and asked: "Are we going to ignore what Marty Mann said, or are we going to do something about it?"

After some conversation, the good sister said: "I tell you what, George. We have a sixteen-bed unit that lies vacant and unused in the hospital. It is now yours to turn into a chemical dependency unit."

Mann was taken aback that her response was so immediate and so practical. Upon leaving the office, he asked himself: "Now what do I do?" He had accepted the challenge even though he had no professional training in addiction medicine. St. Mary's hired the Johnson Institute to create the program, and Mann agreed to be the director.

Refurbishing the unit was going to take about six months, which allowed him some time to plan a program and bring a team together. It had to be a medical model because only doctors could admit to the hospital. But there was no model for a hospital so he had to create one. Hazelden seemed like the logical choice for help. Dan Anderson, the director, had just finished putting the new units together in 1966, and Mann thought Hazelden would be willing to help him and the hospital by sharing its knowledge and expertise. He made two attempts at talking with Hazelden about working together, but for a variety of reasons this never happened. Indeed, it was not until the mid-1970s that Hazelden had a consulting staff experienced enough to design programs for installation in hospitals.

In the meantime, Mann sought help from Vern Johnson, who was just beginning to find his own creative way in the field. The best Johnson could do was recommend some recovering alcoholics to help staff the program. The original Johnson Institute staff was a volunteer lecturer, group leader, and Hazelden graduate. Ironically, this use of nonprofessional volunteers, as a source of mutual sharing, as well as a cost reduction, eventually became an important part of making The Retreat model an affordable alternative to existing treatment models. Thirty years later, that original Johnson Institute volunteer, Terry Troy, became a valued board member of CORP and The Retreat. Just as in the early days under Pat Cronin at Pioneer House two decades earlier, the "recovering staff" was able to model for the patients what recovery was all about, share their own recovery, and instruct them in the meaning of the Twelve Steps. The treatment was very basic and unscientific, and the team learned by doing. It was an exciting time, and despite what Mann called the staff's "bumbling" in seeking to find their way, the patients got well. "We learned from our mistakes and gradually formed a team of professionals and recovering alcoholics," Mann recalled. It was much like the experience of Willmar State Hospital. (See epilogue.) Soon other hospitals in the Twin Cities followed suit.

In the beginning of his venture, Mann gradually began to feel ostracized by his colleagues. For some years, he was not assigned to any of the medical committees and it was hinted that he was a second-class doctor practicing witchcraft instead of medicine. He felt very alone. One day while riding in the elevator with some of his colleagues one of them asked when he was going to come back to the practice of real medicine. (Dan Anderson, president of Hazelden, remembered being looked down upon by other psychologists because of his practice with alcoholics.)

Also in that first decade after the unit opened, Dr. Mann was spending his time going back and forth from the operating room as an anesthesiologist to the chemical dependency center as director of the program, admitting patients and conducting physicals. Finally, he was told by his colleagues that it would have to be one or the other. He went to the president of the hospital and asked if she would hire him solely as the director of the Chemical Dependency Unit. Sister Madonna agreed. However, the best she could do was to hire him at half his salary.

He went home that night and talked it over with his wife, wondering whether and how he could support his large family on such a reduced income. His wife, relishing the strength of her recovery and what it had done for her physically, mentally, and spiritually, said she would get a job, which she did. They determined that their combined incomes would allow them to live well enough and support their large family. Both acknowledged that by living more simply they would still be able to live comfortably on their earnings.

At the hospital, he and his staff survived the unexpected and the unknown and persevered despite some misgivings and setbacks. Over the years, the treatment program was refined, a first-class family program was added based on a Vern Johnson model. An adolescent/young adult program expanded the continuum of care, and the number of beds increased to 120. St. Mary's soon became known as an outstanding treatment program and attracted clientele from throughout the country.

As the programs unfolded, the staff rallied around a mission that was meaningful and shared in the reward of seeing individuals and families heal. It turned out to be an exciting time, a time to explore new ideas and new ventures, a time to embrace what worked and discard what did not. In the early days, the staff was on fire with the gift of recovery, seeking simply to pass it on to others. Treatment was no longer folk medicine, and eventually the whole hospital took pride in the services it provided.

The early 1970s at St. Mary's was an era of simplicity—a simple treatment program that was essentially one of mutual help. The counselors took the leading role and provided the guidance in implementing the recovery protocol: introduction to the fellowship of AA and instruction in living the steps, particularly step one—"the admission of powerlessness and unmanageability." In the beginning, there were no state regulations, no licensure requirements, and no national standards from the Joint Commission on the Accreditation of Hospitals. There were no managed care companies to satisfy in these early years. Looking back, those involved recognized that they had been through a unique, almost utopian, experience. And those exciting, innovative days would never be recaptured. Things were simple. Individuals and families got well, and their gratitude was enduring. Things would change.

First, the growth of the treatment field over two decades was staggering. Along with that growth, the competition for patients was fierce. Some marketing and diagnostic practices became suspect, as filling beds became the overriding preoccupation. As more and more for-profit providers entered the field, quarterly dividends sometimes challenged treatment outcomes as the central concern.

Just as it seemed that the treatment of chemical dependency was gaining respect and confidence, insurance companies expressed their concern at the bills that were being charged to them. They hired companies to manage the reimbursement provided for care. The consolidation, health surveillance, and concentration of control and power that managed care soon exercised had a serious effect on the treatment field. With the introduction of managed care and other variables mentioned in chapter one, eventually the expansive network of treatment that had been built up over two decades slowly began to crumble.

Moreover, treatment was changing at St. Mary's, and according to those who had been on the scene from the beginning, professionalism appeared to be getting in the way of a simple treatment process. Dr. Mann remembered sitting in on staffings where the supervisors would wax eloquent on theories of behavior and how they should be incorporated into the treatment plans. Gradually, mental health staff assumed even larger roles in the treatment process. Mann wondered what had happened to the simple program that had been initiated, founded on the protocol of a fellowship and the kit of spiritual tools—the principles of the Twelve Steps.

Mann retired as the director of St. Mary's chemical dependency program in 1989 (after forty years at the hospital) because he could no longer meet what he knew were his patients' needs under the reimbursement restrictions. He had become a recognized and outstanding leader in the field. He admitted that he was exhausted fighting with managed care for the admission of patients and about the meaning of medical necessity in the case of individual patients. Mann recalled, "As we moved through the decade, the health-care environment became increasingly restrictive and money to pay for treatment began drying up." At the time, he was anxious about what would happen to the whole field.

The field was in a state of serious crisis or, as William White describes it in *Slaying the Dragon: The History of Addiction Treatment and Recovery in America*, "in search of its soul." Occupancy rates for private in-patient treatment programs had plummeted, and more and more hospital units had closed. Precertification and approved reimbursement dropped from twenty-eight days to five-to-seven days, and finally just a few days for detoxification. What followed was a scramble to establish outpatient programs across the United States since managed care would pay for these much less expensive treatment settings.

Mann was convinced that the spiritual principles of AA were at the heart of recovery, and he never lost sight of that vision. He found a kindred spirit in John Curtiss, vice president of Hazelden's National Continuum, who was on his own journey, and would soon be wondering about the direction of the treatment field. He, too, was finding that treatment was becoming overly complicated, less accessible to those who needed it, too expensive and losing its focus on the spiritual principles of recovery.

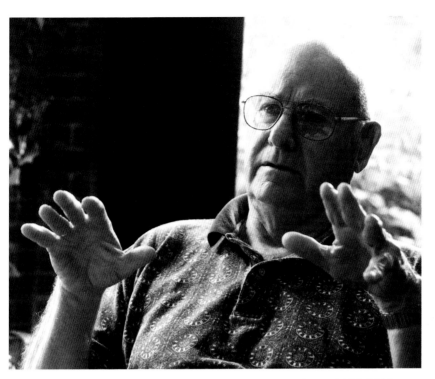

George Mann, founder and chairman of CORP, 1991-2012.

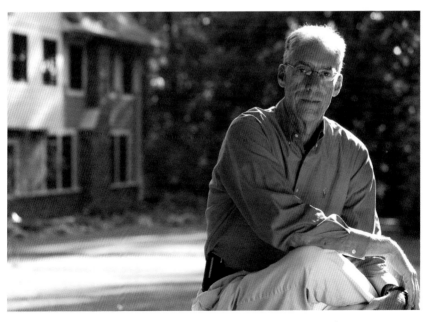

John Curtiss, Retreat co-founder and president.

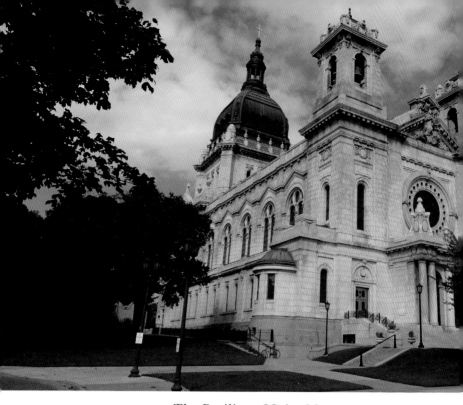

The Basilica of Saint Mary.

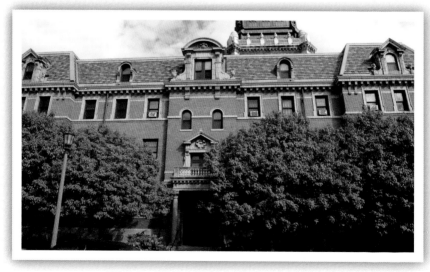

The Basilica of Saint Mary Rectory.

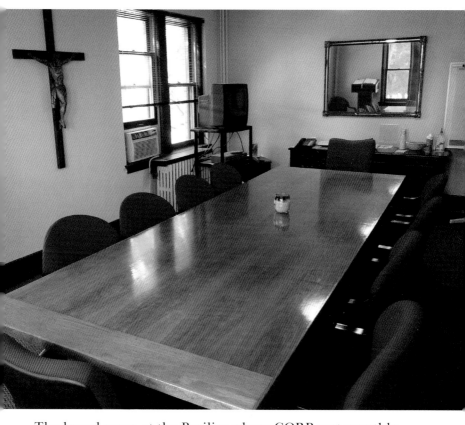

The board room at the Basilica where CORP met monthly for seven years, exploring treatment/recovery options.

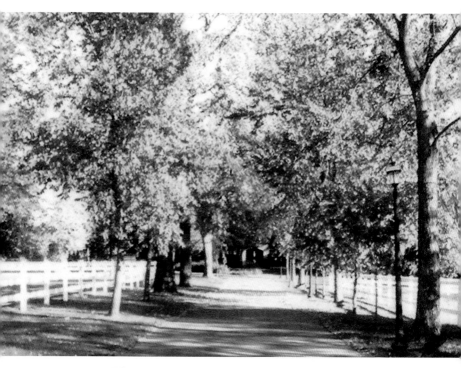

The driveway to The Retreat at Upland Farm.

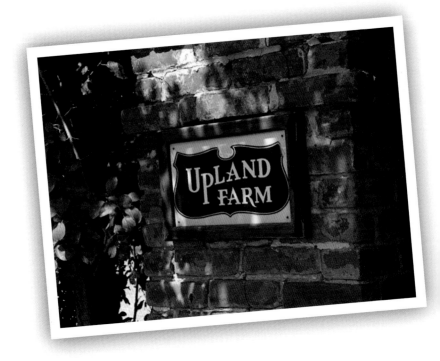

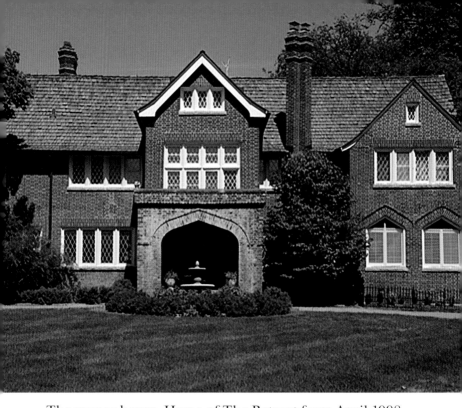

The manor house. Home of The Retreat from April 1998 through September 2004.

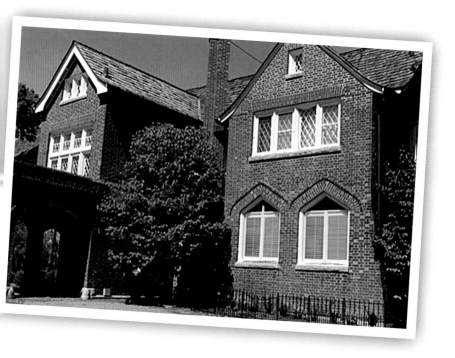

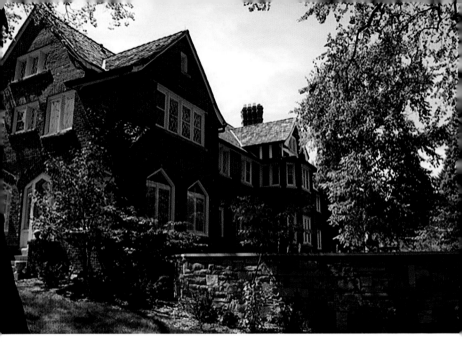

Back view of manor home and patio.

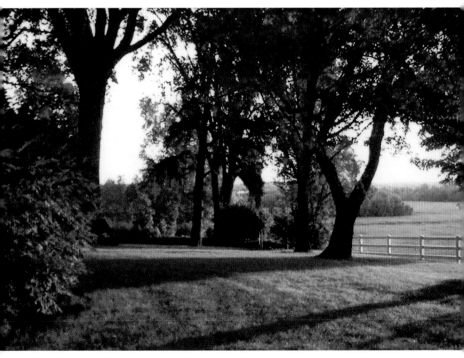

Side yard view of The Retreat's 172-acre Upland Farm property.

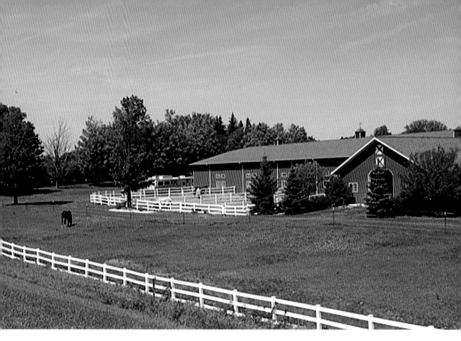

The horse stable and pasture at the
Upland Farm property.

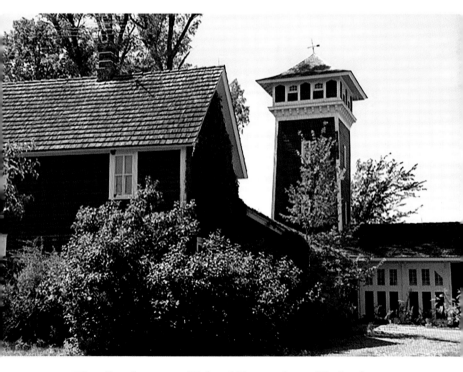

The Gatehouse at Upland Farm where Herb, the
groundskeeper, and his wife lived.

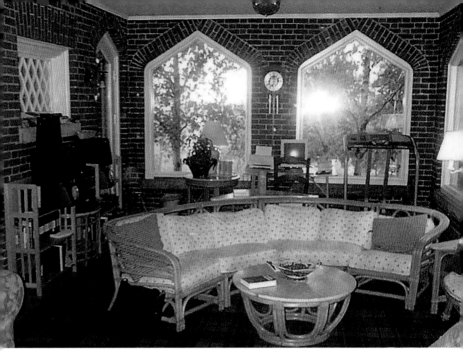

Original wicker furniture in the sunroom where all Retreat meetings were held.

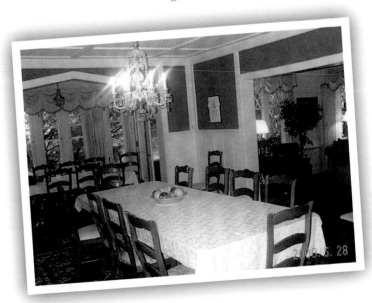

Original Retreat dining room where all staff and guests ate meals together.

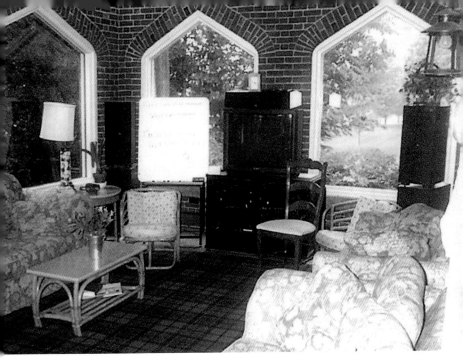

Retreat sunroom where most guest meetings were held.

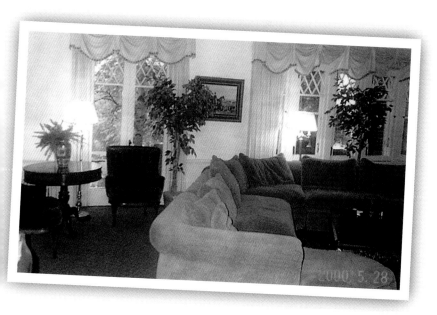

Living room at original Retreat.

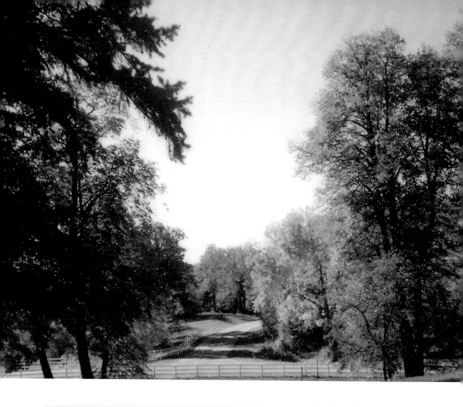

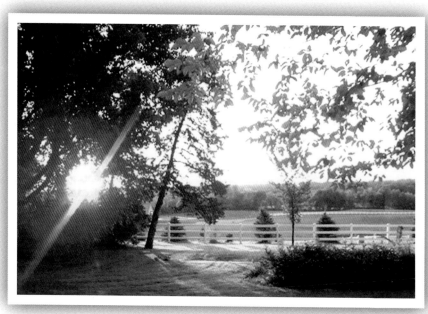

The grounds at the Upland Farm property were beautiful year-round

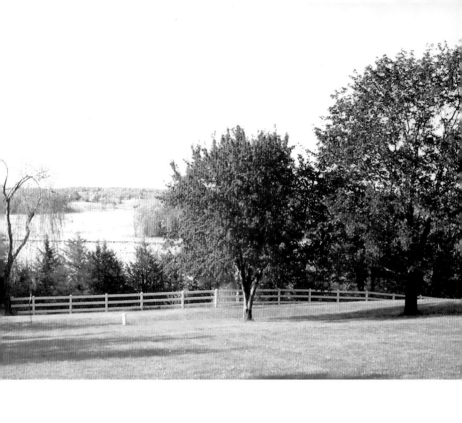
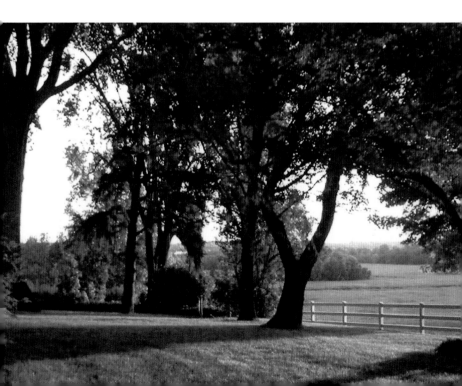

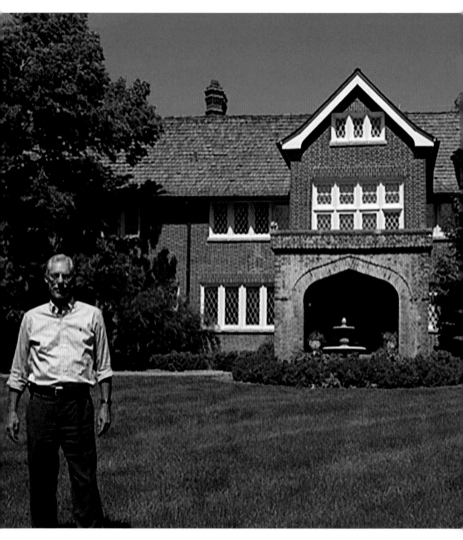

John in front of the manor home.

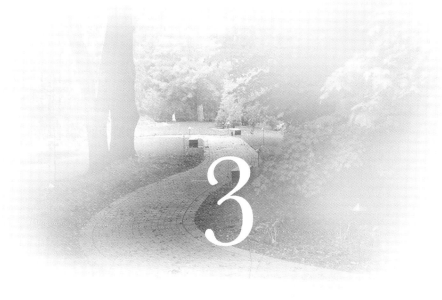

CORP: Community of Recovering People

Minnesota, known as the "Land of 10,000 Lakes," has also been referred to (with tongue in cheek) as the land of 10,000 treatment centers watered by its distinctive model for treatment. In fact, the *New York Times* editorialized about the number of New Yorkers who chose to stay in the recovering community of St. Paul after their treatment. The Retreat has its roots in the Twin Cities of Minneapolis and St. Paul. The men and women who founded The Retreat owe much to the treatment ambience in Minnesota. The dignity and respect for each individual patient emphasized by the Minnesota model, the belief that chemical dependency was a disease, and the sense of community that it sought to create within the framework of treatment all played a role in the thinking and lives of the members of CORP who had previously been involved in chemical dependency treatment for many years.

However disheartened George Mann was by the struggles confronting St. Mary's treatment programs, his determination to help the chemically dependent never wavered. He had thoroughly embraced the spiritual foundation of Alcoholics Anonymous (AA) and how it changed lives. He searched for other outlets for his energy to keep that program alive for those in need. After leaving St. Mary's, he was invited to join the Johnson Institute as one of its directors and continued talking to and sounding out other people as to how best to invest time, talent, and money in helping the chemically dependent.

It was in the context of these conversations and meetings that the seeds for the mission of the Community of Recovering People were sown. All members of CORP played a substantial role in the treatment field or recovery in one way or another. They were displeased and anxious with the way things were emerging in the field to which they had been devoted, and they reacted strongly to the ever increasing fees demanded by the programs, especially in-patient or residential treatment programs, combined with the suffocating restrictions imposed by insurance companies. The money factor and the loss of a simple and direct approach to treatment based upon AA were stripping the Minnesota model of its original simplicity. Most importantly, millions of people were unable to get help.

It was clear that the treatment industry was no longer serving the best interests of alcoholics because of the pressures and restraints exercised by managed care. This group of dedicated professionals and recovering individuals finally decided they were done with talking and were ready to do something about it. They united under the umbrella of the Community of Recovery in June 1991, and then in February 1992 legally incorporated under the title Community of Recovering People (CORP).

Over the course of two decades, the directors came and went, but the evolving dream that bound them together was the vision of helping as many alcoholics and drug addicts as possible, at the least cost possible, with the best care possible, in a center where a spiritually based program of mutual help was the core of the recovery process. CORP wrestled with how to accomplish its mission in a concrete fashion over the next seven years. The first phase ended in frustration and near collapse. Then, with the founders having passed through a critical transition, their journey took them to a second phase where their resolve, creativity, and endurance finished the task.

The directors were interested in strengthening their own recoveries by implementing the twelfth step and carrying the message of recovery to others. CORP remains a nonprofit entity composed of substance abuse professionals, recovering men and women, and community leaders. Directors changed but the commitment remained the same: to provide services that are spiritually based, readily accessible, affordable, and effective. As its thinking evolved, CORP eventually regarded itself as a vehicle for the creation of a new model for assisting people to enter recovery.

The first meeting occurred in June 1991, and its statement of purpose reminded people that the problems of substance abuse continued to destroy lives despite the good treatment that took place in Minnesota. CORP's brochure noted that one fourth of all deaths in the United States annually were related to substance abuse, and the unnecessary health care, extra law enforcement, auto accidents, crime, and lost productivity resulted in costs of $238 billion annually.

As the meetings evolved, one of the principal goals of CORP was to develop services that would be affordable for an individual without the need to be dependent upon a third party or government reimbursement. The directors were all aware through either personal or professional experience that the problem of substance abuse continued to ruin and destroy lives and families. They were also aware that one of the unfortunate outcomes of the current chaos in health care was that treatment was becoming unaffordable for large numbers of people. A new model for entering recovery needed to be developed, one that would be both affordable and available to all who earnestly sought recovery without the cost and complexity imposed by insurance carriers and the medical model as it then existed.

Particularly crucial was the need to inspire a strong sense of community within the recovering population. Everyone recognized that long-term support brought about positive outcomes for those who participated in treatment programs. As a result, CORP intended to provide critically needed aftercare support through weekend retreats both for those who participated in treatment programs and for those who entered recovery on their own. Residential weekend workshops designed primarily for those just entering sobriety appeared to be a good start in laying the foundation of what CORP was about. The topics of these workshops would revolve around the principles contained within the Twelve Steps of AA. The fees were to be reasonable, and funds would be available for those who could not pay the full or partial cost. There was hardly anything revolutionary in this part of its mission, but it would be a safe beginning. The next few years were spent visiting sites that would provide appropriate settings for just such retreats and, at the same time, coming up with topics for the retreat weekends.

To nurture participation in the recovery community, the directors also intended to work toward the development of a residential retreat program in which individuals would have more intensive exposure to the Twelve Steps as a kit of spiritual tools in the recovery process. It would take some years to evolve because of a lack of clarity as to exactly what form this residential program would take, how it would differ radically from the present forms of professional treatment, and how it would differ from programs requiring state licensure. (This last point came up time and again in the meetings.) This part of its mission would take some time to evolve, but when it did, it mapped out a new and revolutionary direction for the treatment of chemical dependency.

In the beginning, there was a lot of energy among the directors as the group met every month, but without much success in finding a location or planning the series of retreats that had been envisioned. One matter that was hardly discussed was where the money would come from to carry out the CORP mission. In April 1993, CORP received news that the Johnson Institute would provide a grant for $200,000 over two years to carry out CORP's mission of developing a new treatment program.

The grant allowed CORP to hire an executive director, James Clayton, to implement the weekend retreat program. It wasn't long before an assistant, Steve Gordon, was hired to present the programs and provide educational seminars for those professionals who might help market the programs. Meanwhile, a series of weekend retreats were scheduled for 1994. But the focus groups (professionals in the field who were invited to provide input) were only sparsely attended, and as the year went on, one weekend retreat after another was cancelled due to lack of interest and participants. The interest of the directors also began to decline, along with their attendance, as the focus remained on weekend retreats with little or no progress toward a radically different approach to treatment.

Sensing this trend, in early 1994 Mann and Clayton clarified for the board members that there would be an evolutionary approach to CORP's mission: a three-year plan that would start with weekend retreats, followed by weekly retreats, and in the final year of the plan the expectation was to have in place an extended retreat program. This was followed by another directive from Mann in August 1994 for Clayton to move in the direction of a residential program. Clayton's response was the plan for a recovery house for those in early recovery whose commitment would be to stay one week. It was still quite far removed from the goal of a radically different and affordable treatment program available for the chemically dependent needing and searching for recovery.

In that same month, the Johnson Institute rescinded its grant for the second year. The withdrawal of what was left of the grant money triggered some serious soul searching. The members of CORP were restless, and the enthusiasm generated at the beginning seemed to be waning. Some of the members thought it was time to disband, believing that the presentation of weekend retreats hardly merited the time and energy that initially guided the organization.

With the end of the grant, Mann realized that some serious decisions had to be made. Weekend retreats were going nowhere, and the idea of a new center for recovery had lain dormant. Two directors jumped into the breach. John Curtiss, who had come on board in 1992, volunteered to work on a draft business plan for a residential program, and Jan Schwarz, vice president of CORP, agreed to assist him.

The years 1994 through 1995 were critical for CORP. Dr. Mann called a meeting to be held at the Loyola Retreat Center, North Oxford, in St. Paul, Minnesota. The agenda was simple but disconcerting: "Should the organization be disbanded? If so, when? Shall we continue? If so, in what manner?" At the meeting, members voiced their sense that the group seemed to have been wandering aimlessly in the desert without any clear focus except for the monthly retreats, which were cancelled due to a lack of attendance. After some very frank discussion and the strong personality and persuasive power of Dr. Mann, the decision was made to continue, but to focus on one part of the mission— namely a center where the chemically dependent would find a spiritual program based on the Twelve Steps that was easily accessible and at minimal cost. CORP was still breathing, but barely.

In December 1994, Schwarz reviewed the past year and directed a spirited discussion around past errors and what was needed to succeed. She reminded the directors that the program to be created needed to be based upon financial realities (precious little thought had been given to who was going to raise money and how they would do it). Plans needed to be modest, not grandiose. The directors needed to be committed to being a working board. Clarity of purpose and a focused mission needed to guide them.

1995 was a transitional year. In February, Mann had to admonish the directors that too many were missing the meetings and not communicating with the board secretary about their absences. He reminded all that the energy of the active members would decline quickly if things were to continue in this fashion.

However, there were also positives to the year. Curtiss presented the draft business plan to the directors in April 1995, produced in collaboration with Schwarz and Bill Rasmussen. An updated version of the business plan was returned in August for the board's review. Meanwhile, Schwarz and Curtiss were working on a marketing plan, an area in which they both had much expertise.

It was in this same year that the board, at the

suggestion of Curtiss, who was beginning to take a much more active role in CORP's affairs, began to look into the program at High Watch Farm in Kent, Connecticut, as a possible model. (High Watch Farm was created by Bill W. and Marty Mann in 1939 as a spiritually oriented retreat center where alcoholics could reside in a safe, caring community and reflect on the AA program.) The director of High Watch Farm was invited to come for a visit to the board in February. After his visit was cancelled, a trip to High Watch Farm by four board directors was scheduled for June. This too was cancelled. However, the contents and schedule of the program were sent to the directors of CORP, and its program and expectations had a definite influence on the board—and particularly on Curtiss's thinking as he continued his work with others on a business and program plan. The High Watch Farm program served as a model for much of what The Retreat eventually became—a supportive, educational, and nonclinical program of mutual help. In 1996, CORP was ready to develop a new modality of care and concentrate on making it a reality.

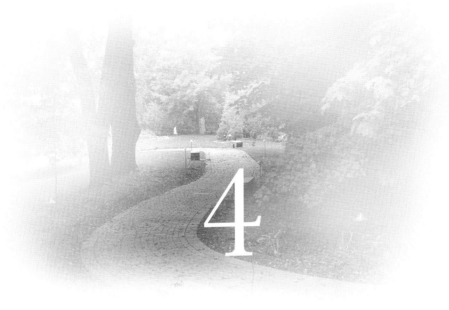

Walking the Road Less Traveled

William White published his monumental work, *Slaying the Dragon*, in 1998, the year The Retreat opened its doors. In it, he clearly outlined the distinction between Alcoholics Anonymous (AA) and treatment, contrasting the difference by describing AA as a mutual help society as compared with professionally directed alcoholism treatment.

In 1996, CORP had found a new direction and an infusion of enthusiasm for the new path on which it found itself walking. The group's energies were directed toward creating something more affordable, innovative, and capable of reaching many more people. From this point forward, the focus would be on fashioning a residential model of recovery based upon spiritual principles and fellowship that would be accessible, affordable, and effective. The crisis was resolved by creating an afford-able model of mutual sharing and a caring community instead of returning to the old paradigm of professional treatment that dominated the field (at a time when these models were very much in decline). CORP had crossed the Rubicon to a new beginning.

The directors agreed to flesh out the idea, contents, and meaning of what would be called "The Retreat" (the name suggested by Curtiss)—a place where people could receive a new set of recovery services that would not break the family bank.

At the beginning of 1996, a new member was added to the board. A successful figure in the world of real estate, Jim Stuebner was a person with high energy and accustomed to getting things done. Then in March, another member of the board, Marlene Qualle, drew up a positioning statement that would keep the board focused. It was a response to the need in the commu-nity/marketplace and differentiated CORP from competitors. This need was for a new model for entering recovery—one that was affordable and available to all. This new program would be committed to establishing services that individuals could afford. The philosophy and spirituality found in the Twelve Steps would serve as the foundation for the program. And the program itself would shift the individual's focus from the rela-tionship with the therapeutic staff to a relationship with the recovering community. As such, The Retreat would provide a bridge between people in early recovery and the recovering community. This growing experience of community would be achieved through the extensive use of volunteers from the recovering community who would serve as speakers, group leaders, role models, and sponsors.

The positioning statement summarized and framed the most important ideas of CORP's mission. The years preceding 1996 were a tapestry filled with a variety of concepts and failed undertakings that served as a prelude to the mission's evolution into a concrete form.

Reflecting upon Qualle's positioning report, Curtiss suggested that the timing was right for the directors to have a retreat for the purpose of reviewing and affirming CORP's goals, objectives, and actions. Stuebner volunteered to host such a meeting at the Northland Inn. The meeting took place on May 13, 1996. Two major items dominated the agenda: a discussion of the business and program plans and a review of the potential locations for the facility.

The program plan provided a tentative road map of what The Retreat would look like, potential staffing patterns, and costs. It called for the development and implementation of a model that would be inexpensive, residential, and educational—not clinical or medical. It described the place as a recovery center, and the program's foundation was to be the spirituality and philosophy of AA's Twelve Steps. A small, experienced staff with the extensive use of volunteers from the recovering community would provide the education and the experience of recovery as well as links to subsequent membership in the Twelve Step recovering community. The goal was to provide a financially accessible, effective alternative to existing treatment options in the Twin Cities metropolitan area, and for that matter, if it evolved, for the rest of the state and perhaps farther. It was later expanded to say that the mission of The Retreat was to not only create this new model of care, but also cause it to be replicated by helping others to find The Retreat model compelling enough to adopt it in other communities around the country and the world. The Retreat model would provide the key elements that were increasingly missing in the treatment field—the gift of time, structure, and support to heal the whole person.

The agenda of the May 1996 meeting also spoke to goals that still needed to be accomplished: fund raising, site selection, facility renovation, state licensing, and community/zoning issues. It was shortly discovered that the projected date of December 1996 for the opening was too ambitious and unrealistic, especially since a location had not yet been settled upon.

Change is an important element of recovery. To live is to change, and to live well is to have changed often. This new model of care would shift the focus of change in an individual's recovery process from the relationship with the therapeutic staff to the relationship with the recovery community. Initially, the program was envisioned as lasting from two to eight weeks. CORP referenced "the sponsorship" and model of High Watch Farms, with over fifty-five years of successful experience in operating a twelve-step recovery program. The executive director would be expected to spend sufficient time at High Watch Farm to better understand the nature of the recovery center and its administrative and program operations. (Curtiss did this in early 1998.)

The plan was for the center to sponsor a rest-and-renewal program for those already in recovery who wished to get back to the basics by immersing themselves in the program and daily routine along with the regular guests.

It was understood from the beginning that the recovery center would not be a substitute for psychotherapy, medical therapy, or detoxification. The program was to have written agreements for services not directly provided by the facility, which would include hospitals, physicians, psychiatrists, and psychologists. The recovery environment was to be pure and simple: an immersion in the spiritual principles of Twelve Steps of Alcoholics Anonymous. (The AA Big Book would become the core curriculum of The Retreat model.)

A committee was given the task of researching and presenting their conclusions at the May meeting. The members of the committee met with individuals in recovery who could share their own personal experiences.

The following benchmarks clearly emerged: sobriety, active participation in the AA community, improved quality of life, and the program's affordability.

At the end of the day, a long list of tasks remained. Among these were securing a facility, formulating a marketing strategy, raising the money to finance the whole endeavor (estimated at about $650,000), and selecting and hiring a director. The business and program plans were tentatively in place. A marketing plan was essential to determine if the community would support such a venture: Would the idea sell with those who were in the position to refer people to the newly created and untested venture? Finding a suitable facility and raising the money to support the venture were other x factors.

It would take a lot of work and perseverance, but after the meeting, there was a great deal of enthusiasm. The members finally had a viable plan that all of them could support and dedicate their time and energies to. George Mann agreed to raise the money, even though he had never raised a single penny in his life. Jan Schwarz would oversee the marketing aspect of the venture.

Having finished the business and program plans, Curtiss and Bob Bisanz were asked to be on the committee looking for a site for the center. Jim Stuebner, a successful real estate entrepreneur, took the lead. Many properties had already been visited, but none of them appeared to fit.

Stuebner introduced them to what seemed an ideal spot in the Western suburbs called Minnetrista, a town of 3,500 people. Stuebner was negotiating with the owners and the banks to buy a large piece of land called Upland Farms, which consisted of 172 acres situated on rolling land with woods, wetlands, and pastures, forty minutes from downtown Minneapolis. He considered the property, valued at $2.1 million, ideal for implementing his idea of an equestrian village. As part of the whole purchase, CORP would be given the potential of leasing 5.2 acres for $72,000 a year with an option to buy at the end of three years for $900,000 (an option that CORP did exercise). Surprisingly, the Minnetrista Town Council had already approved using the manor for twenty guests in December 1996.

Despite some ups and downs in 1997, particularly over negotiations for the property between Stuebner and Curtiss and board member Terry Troy, progress was being made. After meeting with the neighbors for an hour and a half in June 1997, Stuebner sensed there was a concern about the location of a retreat center for recovering alcoholics on the property and he tried to placate those feelings as best he could. Stuebner's bankers expressed similar concerns that interested buyers might not want to build expensive homes on property adjacent to a recovery center; nonetheless, they issued the loan for Stuebner to purchase the large parcel of land.

The opening was set for November 15, 1997, which

proved again to be unrealistic. The money to lease the manor was not there, and Stuebner urged the board to develop a plan to fund the project for about $650,000. Mann regarded himself personally responsible for raising this sum. The marketing plan was still in the works. Initial findings through a telephone survey in June 1997 centering around the need for a program such as The Retreat showed that 37 percent indicated a definite need, 31 percent a possible need, 20 percent a limited need or no need, and 5 percent had no idea. The survey was considered good news.

By the end of 1997, the money had been raised to lease the property. The respondents to the marketing plan questionnaire were cautiously optimistic and consistent in their comments and concerns. They indicated that there was a crack in the current treatment system and the new program seemed to fill that need. It was always helpful to have treatment alternatives.

The big question still remained: Who would direct the program? In one of his earlier communiqués with the board in 1996, Stuebner had already let it be known that it was time to hire a director who could take charge of the venture and bring all of the parts together. In September, Curtiss presented an extensive review of his professional background as a description of what The Retreat would need in any person selected. He felt that The Retreat could be a prototype that could be expanded to other communities. Curtiss would not commit himself to take the position even though he appeared to be the perfect candidate. At the end of 1997, though, he was elected the president of the CORP board. It had been an exciting year, and things were coming together. The money was there, and the property seemed ideal. The marketing plan was in place. But there was still no director. Curtiss continued to feel strong pressure to take the position, particularly from Mann.

Curtiss and Mann's relationship went back to the spring of 1992 when they had met during a conference on Captiva Island in Florida. A two-day meeting brought together professionals from the fields of chemical dependency treatment, research, law enforcement, and other areas and was sponsored by the Johnson Institute. It was a general sharing of experiences related to the present status of the field and ideas about where it might be headed. The discordant note was the disenchantment with the way things had been evolving in the treatment field—particularly the vise-like grip that insurance companies had fastened on treatment programs, the rising cost and complexity of care, and the diminishing access for those in need of services. There was general agreement that the Minnesota model provided good treatment, but needed constant revisiting to maintain its effectiveness and recovery outcomes. Mann and Curtiss were kindred souls who felt strongly and deeply about the spiritual nature of the disease of alcoholism and healing power of the Twelve Steps.

They kept coming back to a common theme: the decline of the field and the fact that there were vast numbers of people in the United States in general and in Minnesota in particular who were not being helped because of insurance restrictions, e.g., medical necessity, preexisting conditions, and the high cost of treatment.

Dr. Mann recalled: "I remember John and I took long walks along the beach sharing a wide range of issues connected with the future of treatment for the chemically dependent in Minnesota: what treatment should be like, what was important and not important. We did agree on the importance of the spiritual experience as the essential core of recovery."

Recovery did not occur by administering the Minnesota Multiphasic Personality Inventory or talking about the effect that parents had on the alcoholic or how someone was raised. They were disheartened by the negative effects managed care had upon treatment during the past decade and talked in general about coming up with a simpler, more basic approach to recovery.

It took some time, but those initial conversations were the seeds of what was to grow into the close relationship between Mann and Curtiss, Mann's invitation for Curtiss to join the CORP board of directors in April 1992 and to assume the responsibility for directing The Retreat as its president in April 1998.

Sober Residences

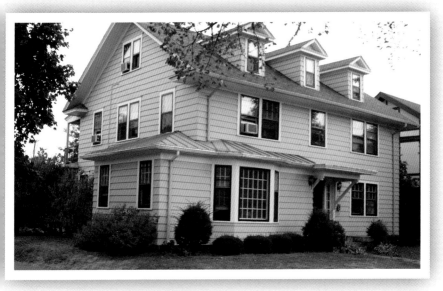

Retreat's first sober house opened in 2000 on
Summit Avenue in St. Paul.

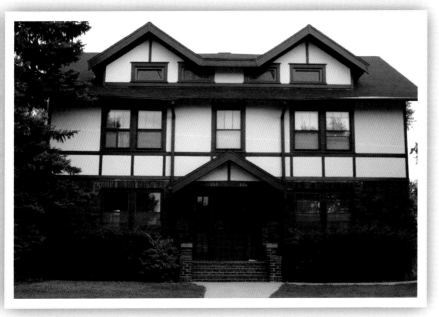

One of 5 Retreat Sober Residence's in the Crocus Hill
area of St. Paul

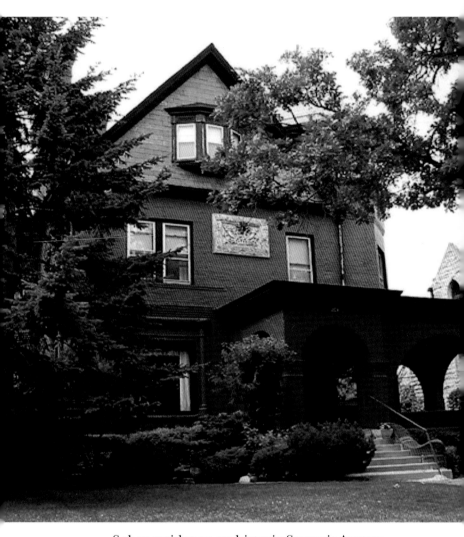
Sober residence on historic Summit Avenue
in St. Paul.

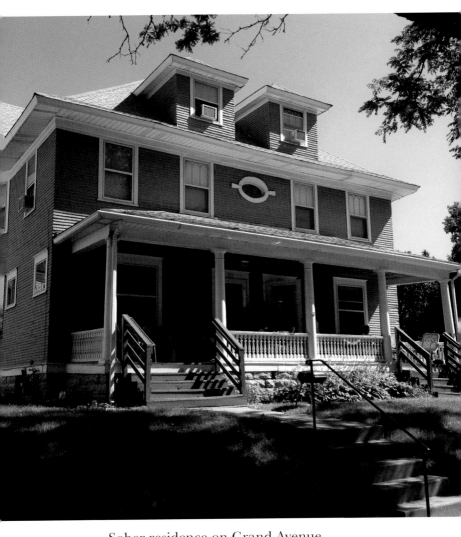

Sober residence on Grand Avenue
in St. Paul.

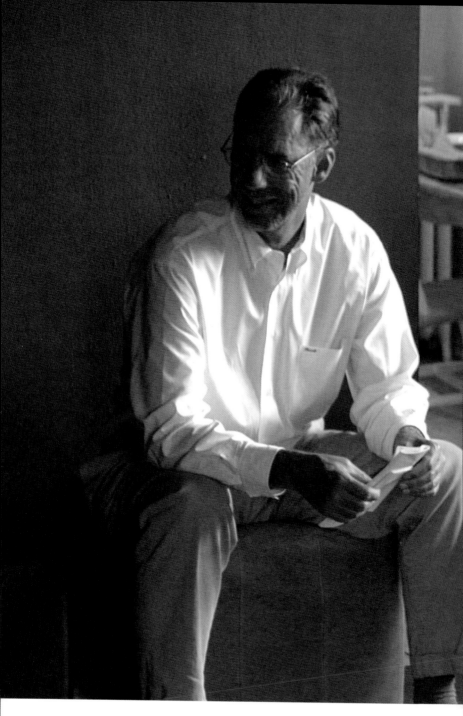

John Curtiss at Tuesday night house meeting/dinner
with the Summit House men.

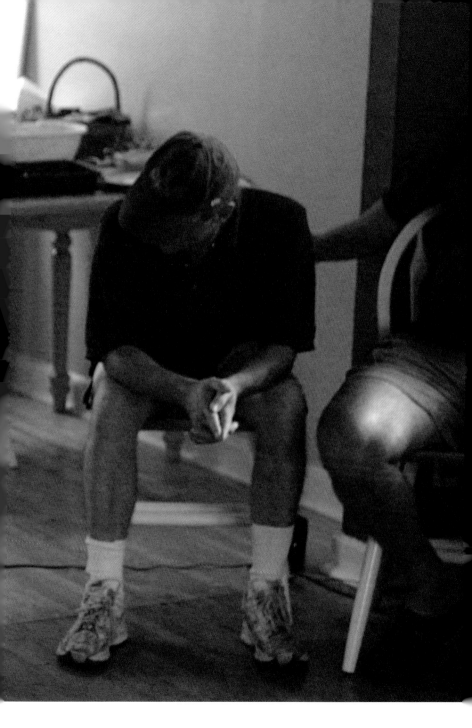

The Cenacle Property

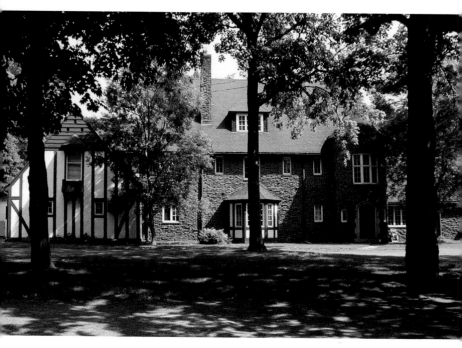

Retreat main building in Wayzata Big Woods.

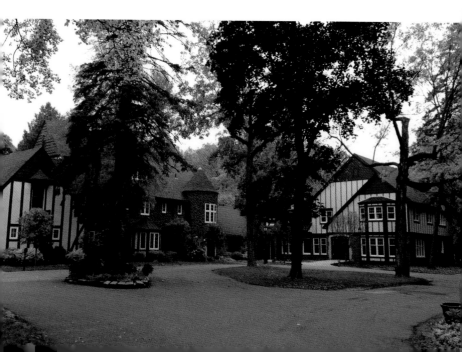

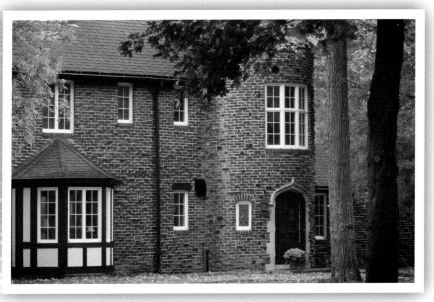

Original Wayzata home built in 1932.

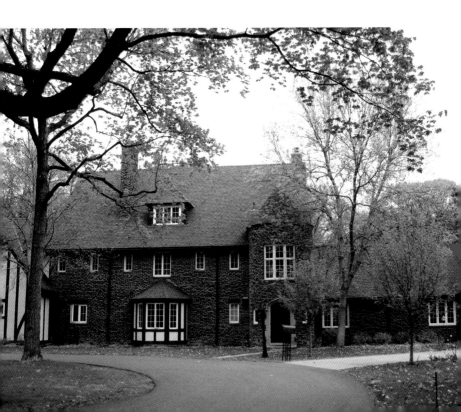

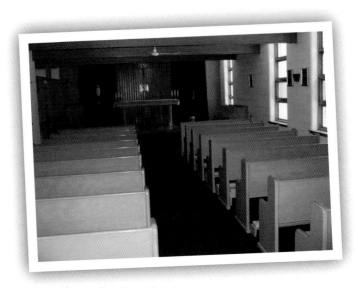

Cenacle chapel prior to renovation, 2004.

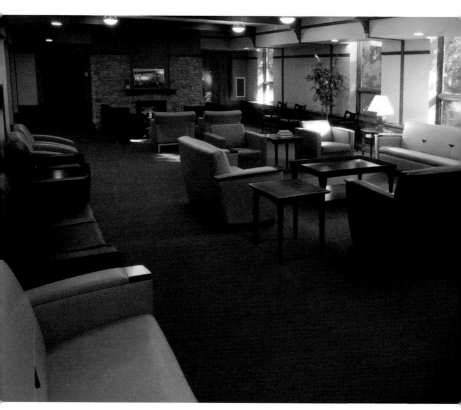

Men's chapel room after renovation, 2004.

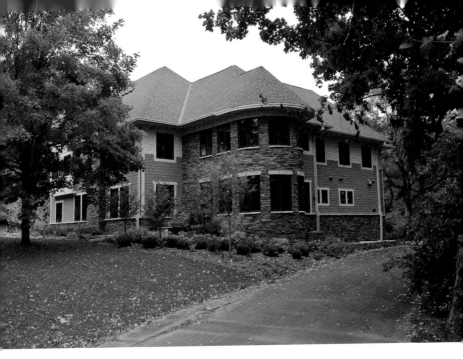

McIver Center for Family and Spiritual Recovery.

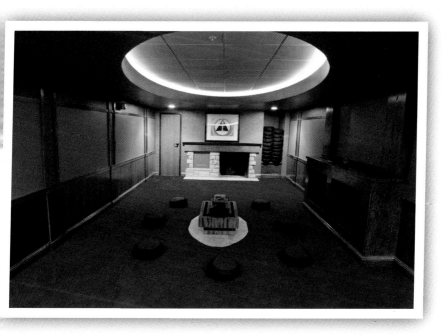

Meditation room.

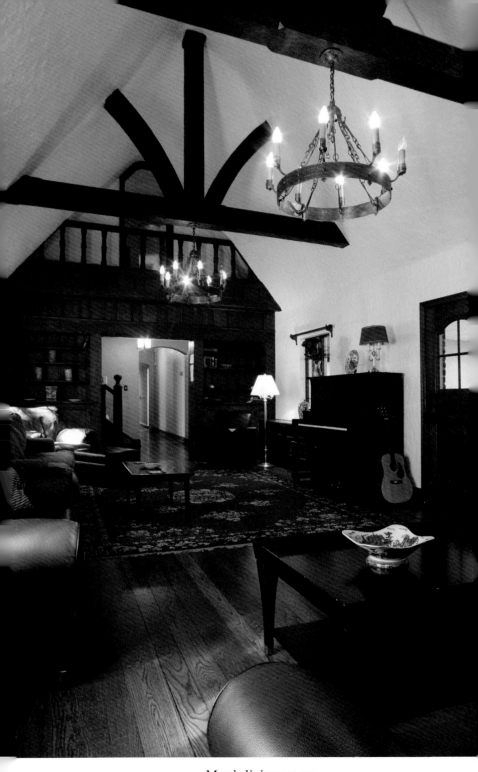

Men's living room.

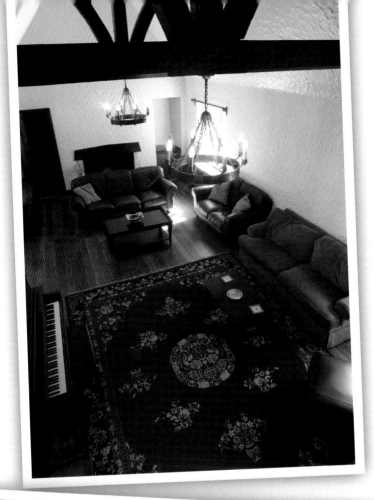
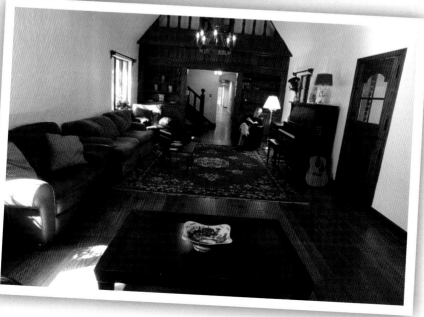

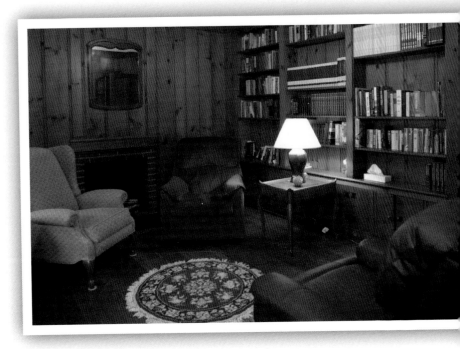

Library where Fifth Steps are heard.

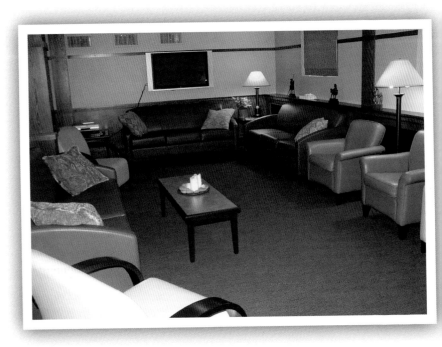

Retreat's Center for Women's Recovery meeting room.

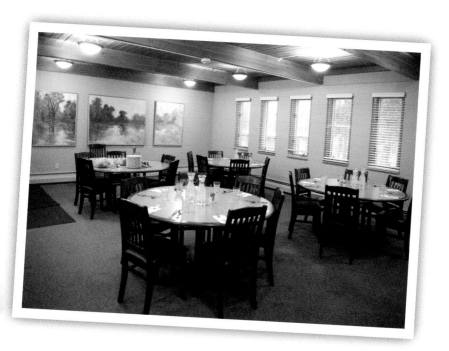

Women's dining room.

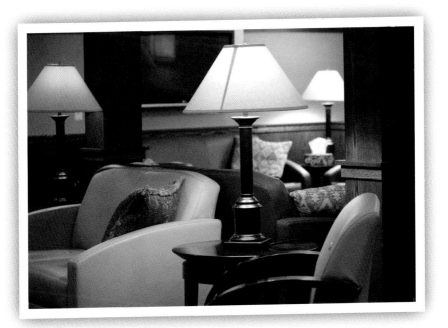

Women's meeting area.

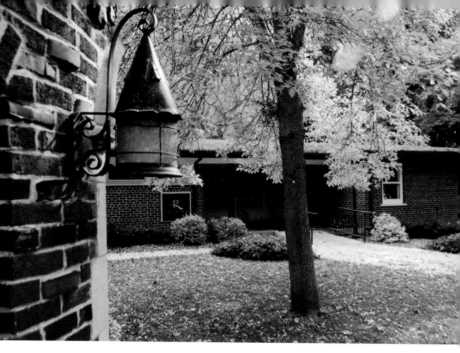

Retreat main entrance prior to two-story addition.

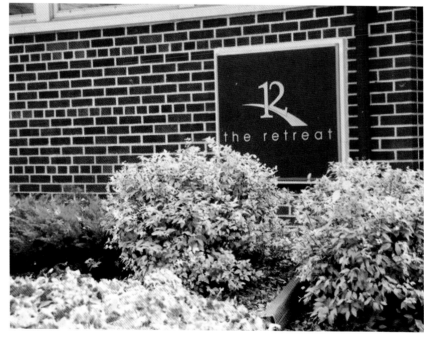

The Retreat R-12 logo signifying its vital connection to the Twelve Steps, a pathway to recovery, the language of the heart, and the humility necessary to stay on the beam.

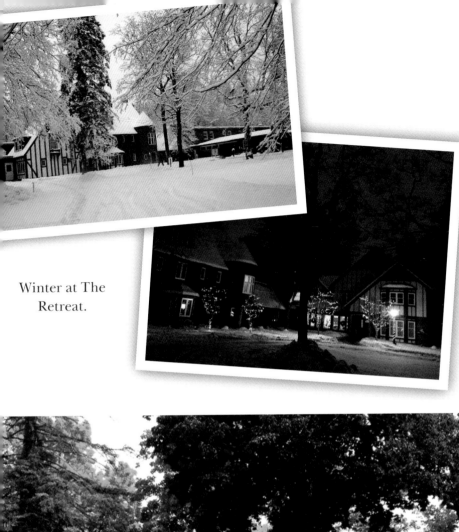

Winter at The Retreat.

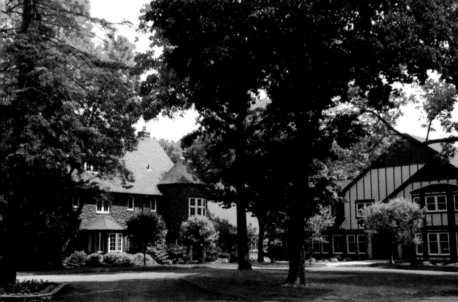

Main building with new addition.

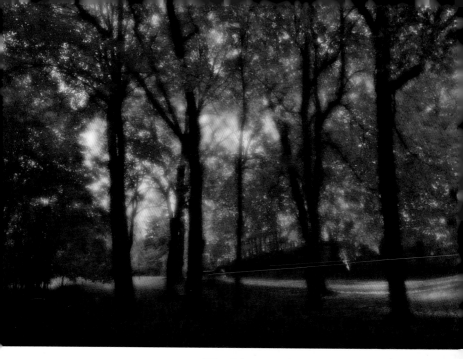

The big woods.

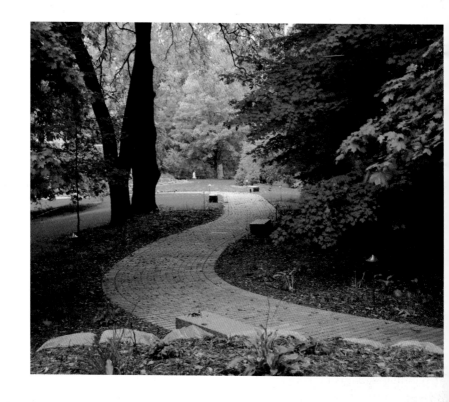

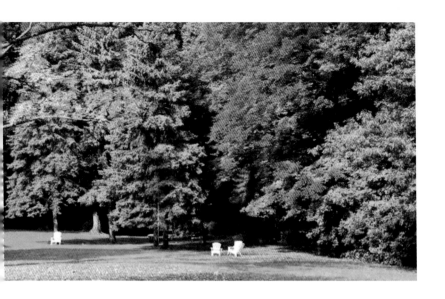

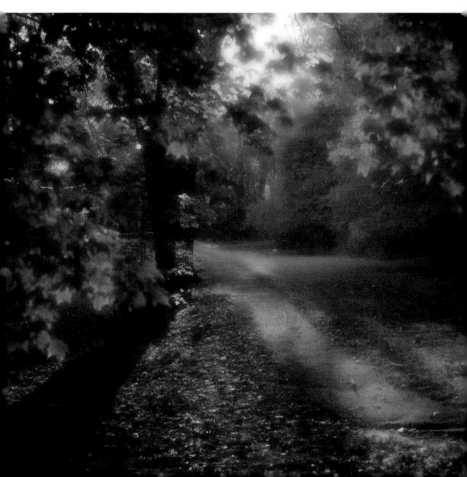

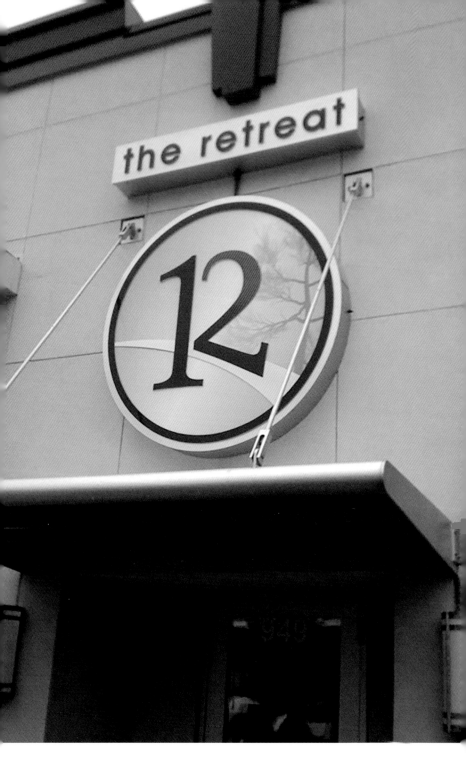

Non-residential office on Grand Avenue.

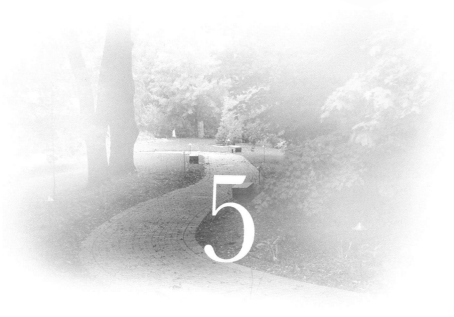

5

John Curtiss, Hazelden

In Curtiss's early years at Hazelden, he came to a fundamental and lifelong understanding of his own personal powerlessness over the illness he had. During those years, he internalized that the answer to his problem of addiction resided in accepting the solution—a power greater than himself and the practice of the Twelve Steps of AA.

The next stage of his education at Hazelden came from his training and subsequent experience as a counselor. He was able to comprehend further the many faces and facets of the disease and how it could conspire to cloak its presence through the art of denial. Curtiss became a fine counselor and, in recognition of his skill, he was promoted to unit supervisor, where he modeled for many the importance of the multidisciplinary team approach necessary in an effective addiction treatment experience. During these years, he came to a deeper understanding of the importance of community, the full continuum of care, and especially the value of the halfway house and sober houses in the role of promoting long-term contented sobriety. He came to fully realize that all recovery-related endeavors had to be based on the spirituality of the Twelve Steps of AA.

His education continued as he began to experience the influence that insurance and managed-care companies were beginning to exercise on the treatment industry and how the treatment centers had to adjust their demands if they were to survive. The means of survival were an ever-increasing reliance on the medical sciences to meet the criteria of medical necessity proposed and defined by the insurance industries as a condition for funding treatment. This accommodation and the systematic changes required by it focused more time on co-occurring issues and diminished the time available to the treatment of the primary illness—chemical dependency. This treatment model was becoming increasingly more expensive and, as a result, insurance reimbursement was fast becoming the customary means of payment for services.

It was now fair game for the critics of the Minnesota model to view its twenty-eight-day treatment program as inflexible and unable to accommodate itself to shorter lengths of stay and the emerging, less expensive outpatient programs.

In the midst of all of these changes, which some have termed "upheavals," Curtiss's postdoctoral education continued when he encountered a group of people who collectively wondered whether treatment could be delivered in a less expensive fashion and reach more people. What he finally learned in the last stage of his education and what together they were able to create was a new model of care that would not be treatment but a caring community—a spiritual program founded on the fundamental principles and Twelve Steps of AA.

As discussed in the appendix, around 1975, Hazelden, one of the principal examples of the Minnesota model, had just completed a decade of amazing activity. The stars had aligned for this little treatment center in Center City, Minnesota, and John Curtiss would soon arrive to begin his ongoing relationship with the center.

On January 2, 1976, Curtiss was provided by his mother and lifelong family friend Dr. David Simon a one-way airline ticket from Cincinnati, Ohio, to Center City, Minnesota, to enter the treatment program at Hazelden. He had already gotten a taste of the fellowship as two AA friends of his father (Chick M. and Gene S.) had been after him for three years, trying to direct him to recovery. They did not desist until he was on the plane. They had made John their mission, and looking back, John had fond memories of how they had surrounded him "with care, love, and their unwavering belief that he could recover in the program and fellow-ship of Alcoholics Anonymous."

When Curtiss arrived in St. Paul, he couldn't believe how much snow was on the ground and how cold it was. He arrived during a major winter storm in which the temperatures plummeted to 30 below zero. When John asked the driver who took him to Hazelden in Center City what the little cabins were doing on the lake, he was told by the driver with tongue in cheek that they were the low-rent district. John found out later that they were the icehouses where the men huddled while they fished through holes drilled into ice that was a foot or more deep. (An unusual sight for a young man from Cincinnati.)

Curtiss arrived at Hazelden a frightened twenty-three-year-old young man who could not imagine living without alcohol and drugs. On Ignatia Hall, the skilled medical unit where he spent his first two nights, he met the head nurse, Dee Smith. She took a special interest in John and assured him that they would slowly taper him off his drugs (alcohol, Valium, and barbiturates). He would not have to go cold turkey, a process he dreaded because he had already been through that a number of times. As it was, it still took twenty-one days before John was fully detoxed. Dee Smith's philosophy was to remove patients from all mood-altering chemicals and replace them with a program of living, a community of support, and the gift of time before determining what their medical/psychological needs would be—a practice that would change in the years to come. John would walk over to Ignatia every day, experiencing muscle spasms and much anxiety. He recollected that it "was not an easy withdrawal."

After Ignatia, he was sent over to the Old Lodge, Hazelden's original facility (which would be closed the following year when the Cronin unit opened in its place). This wonderful, old manor still maintained the closeness, warmth, and charm that the patients had cherished for almost thirty years. At The Retreat's Upland Farm location, Curtiss could not help but compare how the two manors resembled one another with their warmth and an environment in which the guests could feel at home.

Ed Juergens, one of the grand old staff at Hazelden, was his counselor. Juergens provided John with a very simple, yet straightforward, message about the spirituality of change found in the Twelve Steps of AA and gave him daily assurance that he was going to be all right. He was known as a very loving and deeply spiritual counselor who believed in people long before they could believe in themselves. Full group was held in the beautiful dining room. This meeting of all of the patients had had a variety of names over the years. When Curtiss was there, it was called the Hot Seat, where the patient sat in the middle of the circle and was provided loving, serious, and sometimes unpleasant feedback from his peers. These evaluations were written out and handed to him at the end of the session. It was always attended by one or more of the counseling staff and was never allowed to be vindictive, harsh, or disrespectful. It was mutual help at its best. This was the beginning of John coming to believe that he could live a sober, chemical-free life. The experience of hope was slowly coming into his life.

After finishing treatment, he was given a medallion in a closing ceremony surrounded by his peers, indicating that he had successfully completed the program. He was overwhelmed with emotions at the love and care extended to him. He then spent the following month, February, sleeping at the Hazelden motel, a short distance from the Hazelden grounds. He would return to the Hazelden campus in the morning and participate in the schedule during the day at the Old Lodge, and staff would take him to outside AA meetings in the nearby community in the evenings. This was the beginning of his experience of the importance of continuing care (*aftercare* as it was then called) and being loved into recovery. Curtiss recalled: "The staff went out of their way to carry the message of hope and recovery and care for me when I couldn't care for myself."

At the end of February, motivated by a willingness to go to any lengths and take direction from those who knew more about recovery than he did, John moved to Fellowship Club, Hazelden's halfway house in St. Paul, founded by Pat Butler in 1953. There, John had plenty of time to practice his recovery where the principles of AA were lived and internalized in a setting of fellowship and mutual help. He remained there for eight-and-a-half months. (It was this personal experience that convinced Curtiss how important time, structure, and support after treatment was for sustained recovery. It motivated him to quickly establish The Retreat's "residences" for sober living.) This experience was reinforced twelve years later when he became the executive director of Fellowship Club.

Finding and keeping a job was one of the more important requirements of the Fellowship Club. He worked a variety of jobs including shoveling snow, moving furniture, and pumping gas. He developed a good work ethic. When he graduated from Fellowship Club, it was suggested that he move into a sober house to continue surrounding himself with a community of support. His first experience at a sober house was not a healthy one because the other residents sat around watching television all day. He told Dick Feldman, the supervisor at Fellowship Club, that there had to be more to recovery than that. Feldman agreed and made arrangements for him to transfer to another house in St. Paul.

Working every day for Web Publishing for two-and-a-half years strengthened his already strong work ethic. Curtiss associated with a lot of young people in recovery and remembered those years as being great times.

There were a lot of sober dances and sober volleyball and softball leagues. Treatment centers based on the Minnesota model were springing up everywhere. There was this sense of an extended family/large community in the Twin Cities. The Freedom Fest in June 1976, which brought together thousands of recovering people from all over the Midwest to gather at Metropolitan Stadium in Bloomington, Minnesota, in a celebration of recovery, was a testimony to the growth of the Fellowship.

The time came when the job at Web Publishing became boring. Curtiss had come to the point in his life where he wanted to find a greater purpose and meaning in what he was doing. He recalled hearing Sister Marlene Barghini talking on public radio about her shelter for runaway youth, The Bridge. She needed volunteers. He called, interviewed, and was accepted. He spent between twenty and thirty hours a week answering phones, taking kids on walks, and running groups from 3:00 to 10:00 p.m. He also continued to work the 11:00 p.m. to 7:00 a.m. shift at Web Publishing and went to a lot of AA meetings. They were long and tiring days, but he enjoyed working with young people. His long hair, which he shed a few years later, and his empathic heart for working with young people helped him gain acceptance with the adolescents with whom he was working. Curtiss had found a mission in the helping profession.

After a lot of praying, three years of solid sobriety under his belt, and his experience at The Bridge for

Runaway Youth, Curtiss was committed to take the next step on his path to a life of meaning and purpose. He was accepted into Hazelden's counselor training program, a fifty-five-week formal counselor training program initiated in 1975 under the direction of Jake Kenyon (who was succeeded by Dorothy Flynn in 1978). His sleeping accommodations were on the lower floor of the Jellinek unit, which was set apart for the counselor trainees. Curtiss felt as though he had returned home.

Curtiss invested himself completely both in the training program and in the life at Hazelden. Living the twelfth step by carrying the message to others gave meaning and purpose to his life. When he was not studying, going to classes, or working with patients, he was mingling and talking with housekeepers, drivers, cooks, nurses, and switchboard personnel—absorbing the energy found in the total Hazelden community. Walking the hallways and meeting spontaneously with patients became one of his important treatment principles, which he subsequently required of his staff at The Retreat. "Spend less time in your office and more time in the hallway influencing the spirit of community" was Curtiss's mantra. He clearly practiced what he preached. He remembered Dorothy Flynn telling him that "we don't want to train that natural empathetic spirit out of you." However, she knew that he needed a break to discover that there was life outside of Center City.

His experiential training began on the Jellinek

unit, named after E. M. Jellinek, the noted alcoholism researcher at the Yale Center of Alcohol Studies, and continued on the Lilly unit, named after Richard Lilly, who provided the initial funds for the purchase of Hazelden in 1949. His education convinced him that as a counselor treating the chemically dependent person, one comes to know and understand people at a deeper level. Curtiss knew that it was through the language of the heart that he could best help those who were still suffering.

In March 1980, Curtiss began his official career with Hazelden when he was hired as a float counselor, the designation given to staff who were not assigned to a particular unit but instead helped out on any of the six units, wherever the need arose. He remembered carrying a caseload of fifteen patients on three units. Today, because of the workload required by any number of agencies, federal and state, as well as insurance and managed care, counselors at Hazelden carry a caseload of only six or seven patients.

In 1983, he was promoted to the position of unit supervisor responsible for the Cronin unit (named after Pat Cronin, Minnesota's gift to the AA movement). In 1986, he became the unit supervisor of Silkworth (named after Bill W.'s doctor, friend and advisor Silkworth, who wrote the Doctor's Opinion for *Alcoholics Anonymous: The Big Book*.)

At this time, Curtiss began to see the extent to which

external agencies were encroaching upon the care that treatment programs were providing. The explosive growth of administrative requirements and the ever-increasing attention on the medical record consumed more and more time in the counselor's day, short-changing the time available for direct patient care. This started at the end of the 1970s when clinicians had been confronted with the pressures of licensure, certification requirements, and national accreditation standards.

Added to these same regulatory, quality assurance, and licensure demands, the clinicians of the 1980s now had to deal with the insurance companies and managed care, which required dealing with bureaucracies and an ever-increasing amount of paperwork. Throughout it all, they sought to maintain their allegiance to the funda-mentals of the treatment process: patient education of the twelve-step recovery principles through the lecture series, the creation of fellowship through sharing and identification, and the basic clinical services of group meetings and one-on-one counseling. Curtiss developed a reputation for creating enthusiastic multidisciplinary teams with a strong focus on spirituality and the Twelve Steps of AA, a strength that would follow him through his entire career.

Still, in the 1980s some of the older staff began to yearn for the days when their work was uncomplicated by state and national requirements and their mission was clear and simple. They departed, feeling that it wasn't simple or fun anymore. (Ed Juergens, Curtiss's counselor, was a case in point.) Others, the young and eager to whom the old guard had passed on their clinical skills and wisdom, replaced them.

Curtiss remembered one of the striking things that emerged in the 1980s was the quantification principle. Not only did services improve as the team developed and worked with one another but services also multiplied. Eventually the pace became very hectic for the patient as the members of the multidisciplinary team vied with one another for appointments and time with the patients, and the patients began to complain that they did not get to see their counselors often enough.

As the chairperson of the Hazelden's Clinical Staff Organization, Curtiss had firsthand experience of the hours of committee work focusing on and meeting accreditation and licensing standards, and codifying treatment activities in preparation for surveys. Things were getting more and more complicated. Curtiss remembered talking with Dan Anderson before he retired as president of Hazelden in 1986. Despite his position over the years as president, Dan remained very human and caring. But he remarked on a number of occasions that he was worried that Hazelden was getting too big, too complicated, and too expensive, a trend that was happening across the addiction treatment field in the United States.

With the strong role that insurance began to play

in treatment, the question inevitably arose: Who was driving patient care—clinicians or insurance? Moreover, the profiles of the patients were becoming increasingly complicated. It became imperative to match staff professionalism and competencies with the presenting patient profiles. The alcohol and drug abuse clients arriving at Hazelden presented very differently from the patients of one or two decades previous showing up with multiple emotional, mental, and physical health problems in addition to multiple drug problems. In this context, the professional counselors' role had to continually evolve, requiring more education, more specialized skills, and broader knowledge than the professionals before them. The pressure was there to move from the treatment of the chronic disease model to a model that included co-occurring disorders. Physicians, nurses, psychiatrists, and psychologists played an even larger role in the delivery of services for the chemically dependent.

As unit supervisor and later as executive director of Fellowship Club, Curtiss had to deal with managed care and the counties who referred to the halfway house. When he became vice president of Hazelden's National Continuum in 1992, he was confronted with the especially demanding pressures of insurance companies in New York, encounters that were not always pleasant. This was balanced by the excitement of creating Hazelden's fifty-five-bed intermediate-care facility and a vibrant caring community in the United States' largest city.

At first, Hazelden sought to adjust to the managed-care concerns about admissions and the insurance companies' demands for discounts. At one point, the Hazelden leadership said no to the discounted contracts. But that changed after the death of Pat Butler in 1990 when the business members on the Board of Trustees insisted that Hazelden take a more conciliatory tone with the insurance companies. Hazelden also embraced a very active role in the health-care reform spearheaded by Hillary Clinton shortly after Bill Clinton became president in 1992. Unfortunately, the health-care reform failed and hundreds of treatment centers across the United States were forced to close. The remaining centers faced difficulties regarding reimbursement since after the failure of the Clinton initiative insurance companies felt emboldened to continue their opposition to residential treatment and their support for restricted reimbursement.

The implementation of the Minnesota model gradually changed in the 1980s. Some of the change had to do with the loss of the spirit of smallness, some of it had to do with the competition among the multidisciplinary staff for the patient's time, and much of it had to do with the perceived evolving complexity of the patient profile. The counselor's role continued to evolve with the need for more education and more specialized training in the mental health issues and co-occurring disorders. It was in this context that Curtiss returned to college, then on to graduate school where he received an MA in human and health services administration.

Of course, he knew that more degrees did not necessarily mean better care. Indeed, the temptation would arise for the counselors to neglect the soundings of their hearts for the calculations of their intellects. Curtiss worried that the field was "losing its anchor in the language of the heart." He recalls speaking to the president of Hazelden about his fears that treatment was becoming too clinically oriented and losing its foundation in spirituality. The president assured Curtiss that that would never happen.

But clearly the medical model and outside influences were driving the field from the language of the heart to the language of business. What appeared to exemplify this best was in the mental health area. In the early days of Hazelden, only a small percentage of patients presented with mental health issues (now labeled as co-occurring disorders). The part-time psychiatrists and psychologists, at the direction of the counselors, would assess the patients to determine whether they could be successfully treated for chemical dependency and then referred patients to other mental health professionals for treatment of their co-occurring disorders. Otherwise, the patients would be referred out immediately for care for the primary mental health issues.

But a radical change evolved quietly when mental health services assumed a more active leadership role in the treatment-planning process. The requirement of insurance companies that treatment providers document medical necessity to justify admission and reimbursement into residential treatment further drove the field into the mental health paradigm. Hazelden, for example, went from an estimated 17 percent of the patient population being assessed with a dual diagnosis in the 1970s and 1980s to 60–90 percent in the 2000s. Curtiss recalled Dan Anderson saying, "Many presenting psychological issues would disappear with total abstinence from mood-altering chemicals, active involvement in AA, and time"—a luxury that was no longer possible in this current funding and regulatory environment. Some long-time staff witnessing the evolution of the dual disorder paradigm felt as though the field was focusing too much on the assessment and treatment of co-occurring disorders and not enough on teaching the spirituality of change embodied in the Twelve Steps.

The growth of managed care and its requirement for medical necessity made it necessary to render such a diagnosis in order to deliver appropriate treatment to a patient who would otherwise have been refused funding for care. Some even worried that this need to medically justify treatment had the risk of requiring the finding of pathology in order to be able to deliver needed treatment. Due to the pressure applied by managed care to diagnose and treat co-occurring disorders early in the treatment process (frequently within the first week), a much greater number of patients were being labeled and treated for conditions that may disappear with the gift of time, structure, and support. "No one doubts that the complexity of the patients has increased over the years, but clearly the pendulum has swung the other way," Curtiss said. The unintended consequence of this funding model dramatically increased the cost of care and further diminished access to treatment.

Curtiss was aware of another troubling trend. He clearly saw that the multiplication of services was putting the patients into a time crunch and forcing the professionals to vie for the patients' ever-diminishing slots of free time. Acuity and complexity were growing at exponential rates. Acuity referenced the extent and severity of the patient's pathology and the complications associated with it. Complexity referred to the ever-increasing number of services needed to care appropriately. The cycle of a growing and empowered number of psychological staff and increasing mental health diagnoses and treatment inevitably drove the cost of treatment up. There seemed to be little anyone could do to escape the formula that as acuity increased so did complexity and cost, which ultimately reduced access to care. Curtiss wondered where it would all end because it was becoming more expensive to run inpatient programs. Hazelden was founded in 1949, in part, to remove alcoholics from the psychiatric hospitals where outcomes were poor and hopelessness prevailed. Instead, they were to be welcomed into a dignified caring twelve-step community retreat environment where one could find recovery through mutual help. Now the field was being driven back under the umbrella of psychiatry.

The first half of the 1990s were not easy years for the treatment industry as treatment centers across the United States continued to close. The people Curtiss had admired and loved were passing from the scene. Pat Butler, with whom Curtiss met with once a week at Fellowship Club, died in 1990; Dan Anderson was no longer active, although he continued as a board member; and Harry Swift resigned in 1991.

Curtiss was feeling that a simpler, more basic, and affordable approach was needed to help alcoholics recover. In 1995, CORP had been rejuvenated and was now purposeful in its direction for a residential center. Having been one of the directors of CORP since 1992, Curtiss committed himself in 1995 to a more active role in its affairs. In doing so, he entered a critical transition period and went from a passive participant in the affairs of CORP to an active participant in the meetings and the efforts to create something new in the chemical dependency field. (See chapter 4.)

He soon began to feel a subtle pressure to participate full time in the CORP operation, which he knew meant leaving Hazelden. He had already enjoyed a long and successful career there and had a great love for the institution that had saved his life and the work that it had done and continued to do in the treatment field. He was nonetheless becoming truly disenchanted by the changes in the treatment field—the subtle temptation to forget that chemical dependency was the primary illness requiring a spiritual solution.

Administrative tasks consumed more of Curtiss's time. The era of Total Quality Management (TQM) excited the board and senior management. Curtiss was witness to the initiation of process-improvement teams, which became very time consuming. This focus on TQM appeared to weigh the organization down. One of the ends of TQM was to increase confidence and drive fear out the front door. At the same time, real fear was coming in the back door because Hazelden, like the rest of the field, found it necessary to downsize in the early 1990s.

All of these changes made Curtiss restless and uneasy. The great treatment center, along with the field, did not seem to be on the right path. He felt that the direction of the Minnesota model was no longer consistent with his own values. It was painful for Curtiss to come to this decision. Every role that he had served at Hazelden had been the best that he could have wished for. But changes in leadership, combined with his concern for the over-pathologizing of the treatment process and emphasizing business over the language of the heart, weighed heavily on his spirit.

The months leading up to April 1998, when Curtiss resigned from Hazelden, were a time of grieving as he wrestled with the angel of change. It would be a great loss, but he knew that he would have to leave. (He also believed deeply that a change was needed in the field and this was the time to make it happen.) Indeed, once he left and made the transition to a new beginning he never looked back, nor did he regret taking this new path. Curtiss came on board as president of CORP and The Retreat on April 1, 1998. All of the members of CORP were pleased with his decision because they truly believed that they had the best person to implement their plans. George Mann was delighted.

Mann and Curtiss had become very close since their 1992 meeting on Captiva Island, where they had discussed at great length and with much feeling the limitations of the current treatment model and the fact that only a small percentage of those needing help were able to receive it. Their friendship would continue to solidify over the next two decades. Indeed, it is quite likely that without their shared experience of the problems and their shared vision for a new future, The Retreat might never have come into existence.

Under Mann's and Curtiss's leadership and the guidance of other staff and directors, CORP was able to accomplish some truly unique things that stand out in the long history of the treatment and recovery movement. While writing the business plan in 1995, Curtiss came up with the name The Retreat, which was intended to make a statement that this new model was not treatment, but rather a spiritually based, supportive, and educational retreat approach to helping alcoholics recover. This seemingly simple, but profound, shift enabled an escape from the insurance-based, medical model, and added an even bigger benefit. By being grounded in the spiritually based, relational model of mutual sharing and the huge volunteer network that followed, Curtiss added not only enormous cost savings, but also the essence of the caring community, which was at the heart of this new model for recovery.

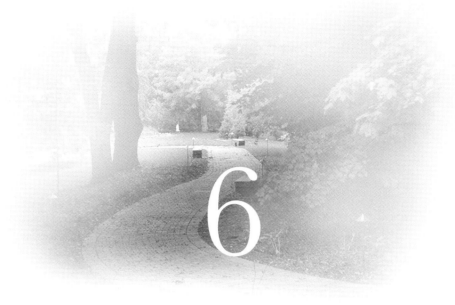

6

The Retreat at Upland Farms

John Curtiss took very little time to put the program in place. The target date for the opening was June 1998, only two and a half months after he came on board, and there was a great deal to be done before that could happen. Curtiss drew confidence from the drive up to the newly leased Manor at Upland Farm—it reminded him of the mile-long drive he had taken to the Hazelden campus under the canopy of the magnificent pines for the past nineteen years. But for all that environmental resemblance, the programs were vastly dissimilar in reaching for the same goal—recovery from alcoholism and drug dependency. He had a clear idea of the program he wanted to initiate, relying upon a caring community and mutual help and not treatment professionals.

That clarity of purpose was reinforced by a visit to High Watch Farm in Kent, Connecticut, for five days in the spring of 1998. Curtiss participated in the program to the extent that an observer was permitted. In reporting back to the CORP members, he described the program as teaching the spiritual principles of recovery embodied in the Alcoholics Anonymous (AA) Big Book, thus carrying on the tradition of Bill W. and Marty Mann. Curtiss found the visit helpful in thinking through The Retreat model and reinforcing what he and George Mann wanted to implement: moving the treatment of alcoholism/chemical dependency out of the traditional medical model and health-care system and into a supportive, educational, community-based retreat-like model of care. They believed that if people could be provided with a safe, supportive environment, accurate information about the problem and solution, and a solid bridge to AA, they would recover.

The core of The Retreat was to be based on a community of peers helping one another. It would provide a safe, supportive peer group and strong linkages to the twelve-step recovering community. Those inquiring about the program with more serious clinical needs would be referred to local treatment, mental health, or medical professionals. The program was designed for a specific target population: those who needed a safe and supportive environment away from the burning house of their addiction, but did not require the clinical intensity offered in a residential treatment program. Curtiss envisioned The Retreat as serving people who knew they had the problem of alcoholism or drug dependency, were motivated for change, and were free from any primary mental health problems.

Dr. Mann believed that the bottom line was that they were starting The Retreat as a living laboratory, as another modality of care that could help more people recover: "We simply recognize that an illness as complex as addiction to chemicals requires constant innovation and creative ways to make care effective and available to more people."

While for Curtiss the clarity of vision for the program was there from the beginning, it was less clear how he was going to manage the preparations and the environment of care. He did have a building. Situated on the center of the property that had been leased and later purchased by CORP was a brick and stone Tudor-style manor of some 8,000 square feet. Driving up to the entrance under the canopy of trees provided one with the sense of moving into another dimension, while leaving the hustle and bustle of the activities of the other world behind. The analogy might be that of entering a sanctuary in which strength would be given and received in a circle of recovering people.

While the building was a great start, it was completely unfurnished and the number of bathrooms, while sufficient, was not ideal. A friend from Hazelden, Gay

Parker, took it upon herself to assist John with the task of designing the use of the rooms and finding appropriate furnishings, the cost for which was equally divided between donations and purchases. Curtiss provided two pieces of furniture symbolic of his past. He was the recipient of the long dining table that had once graced David and Gretchen B.'s home in St. Paul, a special sanctuary for recovering people. He also possessed the rug from the dining room in the Old Lodge at Hazelden, which had closed in 1977 and been torn down in 1987. Its furnishings and antiquities spread to the four corners of staff homes.

Along with the furnishings was the more pressing need of gathering a staff. People were not pieces of furniture whose size, shape, and color could be arranged in a harmonious fashion. However, Curtiss could not have been more pleased with the original contingent of five people.

Misha Quill came on board as the admissions and business office coordinator. Besides being a genius at putting all the necessary forms together for the program, she was a person whose smile could light up a room and whose personality put all of the nervous guests at ease the first time they met her. According to Curtiss, "Misha's warmth and understanding helped define the caring community nature of The Retreat."

Greg Olson was hired as the house manager, a very important position and one of the most demanding.

He lived at The Retreat and accepted the challenge of keeping good order among the guests, who could be unruly at times. The people were guests who could remain or leave as they saw fit—no one was forced either way. Greg had a solid understanding of recovery, which helped him through the good times with the guests who wanted to recover and the difficult times with the more challenging individuals simply going through the motions. He was willing to do anything for The Retreat and its guests.

Diane Poole found a place at the beginning of June. The circumstances were a bit unusual. She had been recommended for an interview by Curtiss's friend, his classmate when they went through training at Hazelden. Curtiss remembered that for all practical purposes it was to be a courtesy interview for he already had his mind set for the position of coordinator of the program. It was an important placement. Whoever filled it had to be of the same mind as the president in forging the new program and its foundational philosophy.

Diane had gone through the Hazelden Counselor Training Program in 1977, two years before Curtiss. She directed Marty Mann Halfway House for women in Duluth, Minnesota, and spent thirteen years of her career working for managed-care companies, a world that she knew very well, but of which she was not the least bit enamored. They both understood the dark side of managed care. She and John conversed for two hours, and it became clear that they were both on the same page when it came to recovery. Curtiss reflected, "Diane was a true professional with an amazing heart for helping alcoholics." She was hired as the program coordinator to supervise the day-to-day activities of the program. The Retreat owes much to the original staff who believed in what they were doing but nonetheless were uncertain as to how the path would unfold.

Joe was the very talented chef with whom the guests felt very much at home. He had great listening skills and was a superb chef with excellent cuisine presentations.

Herb, who lived in the Gate House with his wife, was the groundskeeper. He had a great love and respect for the guests and manicured the grounds with care and skill and helped maintain an environment pleasing both to the eye and enhancing the meditation.

By the end of June 1998, Curtiss had a beautiful and welcoming home and an empathetic, highly skilled staff. Moreover, before The Retreat admitted its first guest it had the seedlings of a committed group of AA volunteers who grew into the corps of recovering people who would make twelve-step immersion come to life. They were essential in fashioning the program into a spiritual retreat—a setting of mutual help, rather than a treatment program conducted and served by a body of professionals.

From the very beginning, the volunteers, under the direction and guidance of the assigned champions, turned out to be an amazingly dedicated and adept group of men and women who had previously had their own spiritual awakenings and sought to carry the message of hope and recovery to others. They captured the spirit of the earlier AA men who were upset that Bill W. would think of taking a salary to talk to other alcoholics. The volunteers became the heart of the program. What motivated staff and volunteers was a sense of doing something new, unique, and inspiring. People drew energy from one another, not always certain that what they were doing would make a difference. But in the last analysis, what they were engaged in was for their own individual recovery. People came and went, but the spiritual energy remained and the traditions were passed on.

Curtiss, with input and recommendations from the Board, was dismantling the accepted treatment model, which relied upon on-campus professionals, and replacing it with a willing and experienced AA and Al-Anon community of volunteers. Why and how this came about can be described as either providence or fate or meaningful synchronicity, depending upon the nature of one's Higher Power.

Here is one example among many. Before The Retreat enterprise opened, Bob Bisanz, another totally engaged and committed CORP director who played a key role in the evolution of The Retreat, urged Curtiss to meet with Chuck R., a recovering alcoholic of many years from the Minneapolis area. At the end of their long conversation, he offered to coordinate an AA volunteer network to transport the guests to AA meetings. This same group volunteered to conduct in-house AA meetings three nights a week as well as to drive the guests to outside meetings another three nights. Essential to the smooth running of these very important services were the coordinators, or *champions* as they were eventually called. Chuck R. and the other coordinators he enlisted were extremely important in fashioning The Retreat into a real and viable mutual service model that could trace itself back to the beginning of AA.

At about the same time, Curtiss met with Roger Bruner (who had the reputation of being a gifted teacher of the *Alcoholics Anonymous: Big Book*) for several hours on the sun porch. They had to make do with the rattan porch chairs before the place had any furniture. They discussed how a series of lectures and discussions on the Big Book could be crafted into a three-week curriculum for the guests. They agreed it would cover the first 164 pages in *Alcoholics Anonymous: Big Book*, from the "Doctor's Opinion" through chapter 7. Curtiss inserted it into the program, and it remained that way. Roger remains one of The Retreat's most cherished champions.

Ellie Hyatt championed The Retreat's Family Day on Sundays, where family members were invited to lunch and an Al-Anon speaker meeting. Marc Hertz championed meditation classes on Thursdays, and

Chris S. championed a fourth-and tenth-step workshop on Saturdays.

Another very important volunteer from the beginning was DJ (Duane Jackson), lovingly referred to as the "spiritual sage" of The Retreat. A great fan of the well-known Trappist Thomas Merton, he came to The Retreat on weekends providing his insights into the Twelve Steps, particularly step three and other spirituality-oriented subjects. Every visit was accompanied by his seeds of contemplation. Scattered throughout the buildings are little signs and sayings, reminders of the spiritual foundations of the program. Besides his talks, he brought with him a little gift for the guests, such as engraved walking sticks and calling cards with spiritual messages, which he had reflected on the week before. Fourteen years later, he remained a weekly spiritual companion and traveler of the program. His traditions as well as the others established in the early years of The Retreat have been extremely important for the growth and life of the community.

The Retreat opened on June 21, 1998. The place was ready, welcoming, and attractive, nothing rich or fancy, but dignified and comfortable. The admission requirements were few and simple. The guest had to be eighteen years or older, sober, and drug free at the time of admission. The guest was expected to be willing and motivated to participate in the program and be mentally and physically capable of meeting personal needs. It was clearly understood that The Retreat's environment and services were not a substitute for psychotherapy, medical or clinical treatment, or detoxification.

The program was to be a supportive and educational caring community based upon a simple formula: active attendance at AA meetings, assigned chores, the study of the *Alcoholics Anonymous: Big Book* and the Twelve Steps and mutual and personal reflections. It was to serve as a bridge to the twelve-step recovering community.

The building was ready, and the staff was in place. The question that had everyone on pins and needles was: Would anyone come? One admission came that first day, Jimmy P., from West Palm Beach, Florida. John had been Jimmy's counselor at Hazelden sixteen years earlier. The relief was palpable. He was surrounded, practically smothered, with attention and care. All of the staff, including John and Diane, attended all of the classes. In those first few weeks, there were more staff than guests. The second guest to arrive, referred by Hazelden, was found to have a hatchet in his suitcase. This was the beginning of many odd experiences that occurred during those first months. The challenges were new, and the responses most often spur of the moment. The exterminator had to be called in for the mice that roamed the basement, and the foundation walls had to be sealed to keep out the small garden snakes that frightened both staff and guests. Jimmy, who loved to drive the tractor, would help Herb cut the acres of lawn during his free time. One guest, who decided to leave the program, packed his bags and started hitchhiking home. He was eventually picked up by an AA member on his way to a meeting. After they went to the meeting together, the AA member brought the guest back to The Retreat.

The underpinnings and spirit of the program were put in place very deliberately and with conscious attention to detail. Fundamentally, what guided the thinking and planning was that The Retreat was not a treatment program. Curtiss was conscious and firm about moving from the hierarchical to the relational, from the professional to mutual sharing. He wanted The Retreat to continuously provide the same feeling of peace and tranquility the guest initially experienced coming up the driveway. As Diane put it, the staff wanted "to love people into sobriety." To promote the spirit of family, the staff, volunteers, and guests all dined together, a practice that continued.

John and Diane evolved a protocol that would create a caring community and dismantle the treatment model of its jargon and nonessential services. The retreat protocol would speak a language of mutuality and caring. The recovery plan would replace the treatment plan. Rather than *patients* and *clients*, residents would now be referred to as *retreat guests*. Retreat would be substituted for treatment, and instead of offering a program, The Retreat would create a caring environment and community. Counseling would be replaced by the sharing of experience, strength, and hope, and a session would simply be a chat with guests in which mutual sharing supported by trust and honesty would occur.

Initially, Curtiss felt The Retreat would be open to everyone who sought admission to the program, but he soon recognized the limitation of his model due to the wide variety of people seeking out The Retreat. Still, the agnostic, the control drinker, and the relapser all found a place at The Retreat. Those who needed more clinical attention were referred to more clinically or medically oriented treatment programs, such as Hazelden or Fairview. Some of the first guests who arrived were in need of detox; they were sent to The Mission Care Detox in Plymouth. Curtiss and the staff quickly developed a network of outside professionals to whom the guests could be sent when an emergency arose or when they needed special medical or mental health care. In short, Curtiss was creating a powerful alternative to the Minnesota model of on-campus professional people—nurses, physicians, psychologists, and psychiatrists prepared to deal with co-occurring disorders and medical issues. In place of the professional counselors, he engaged a willing and tested AA and Al-Anon community and a network of clinicians and therapists in the community who could provide a parallel path of clinical services for those who needed it. The direct agent of change in this model was moved from the counselor–patient relationship to God working through a community of volunteers.

In November 1998, some months after opening, the Minnesota Department of Human Services, in response to a complaint that The Retreat was not a licensed treatment center, visited with Curtiss, the staff, and the guests; looked over the building; and inquired about The Retreat's program. John reported that the surveyor found that a treatment license would not be needed as long as The Retreat did not present itself as a treatment program, did not provide counseling services, and did not take people who really needed a clinical treatment experience. The Retreat, from its inception, chose to license itself as a board-and-lodging program rather than a clinical treatment program, which became a fundamental difference between this mutual help approach and medical-model treatment. That important distinction released The Retreat from the expense and complexity of the medical model. The mutual-sharing model, powered by hundreds of dedicated volunteers, added additional cost savings and supplied and exhibited loving service as an important part of this new retreat-recovery approach.

Given his experience with the importance of family recovery, Curtiss made sure that a simple family experience was incorporated into the mutual help tradition from the beginning. Families, significant others, and friends would visit on Sundays and dine together at the main table with the guests and staff. Children and pets were welcome, and their presence helped create a wholesome and familial atmosphere. Some Sundays, it was more than a bit crowded and gradually adjustments had to be made, but in the beginning all were made to feel welcome.

The plan was that in the afternoon there would be a talk directed toward the families and significant others about the disease and the Al-Anon response. Diane and Roger B. had been talking with Ellie Hyatt, a friend who had much knowledge of the importance of Al-Anon. She agreed to organize a Sunday afternoon session for the guests and their visitors. She acted as the family volunteer co-coordinator (champion) whose role was to contact potential speakers and establish the expectations for the speakers and their presentations. She encouraged the speakers to share their experiences, especially the effect of chemical dependency on family, friends, and significant others. Started at Upland Farms, this Sunday afternoon experience continues with great success to this day at The Retreat.

Essentially, the Al-Anon speakers presented their stories about their relationships with the chemically dependent person, stressing that the solution to the problem could be found in the principles of Al-Anon. The presentation allowed those present the opportunity to identify silently with the experience of others, opening paths for their own recovery through the mutual sharing of strength and hope. The meeting was intended to educate the audience that they were not the cause of alcoholism, that they could not control it, nor could they cure it. They learned that alcoholism is a family disease and that addictive drinking and using affects not only the users but also all of their relationships. Some of the audience were ready to hear the message, and some were not. But the seeds were planted for many of the attendants, and when the pain became severe enough they might finally recognize the direction they had to take, turning to the comfort and strength of meetings, sponsors, and the God of their understanding.

Sundays took on the nature of a big family gathering at which stories were shared, broken hearts began mending, and the beginning of a new life was available to those who would honestly reach for it. Besides playing significant roles in raising money for guest aid, the directors of CORP volunteered on Sundays to share with the families and talk with the guests. Fully conscious of the good work The Retreat was doing and the need for more financial aid, Curtiss hired Bruce Binger as vice president of development, who would play a significant role in the coming years in keeping The Retreat financially healthy.

CORP Board Members

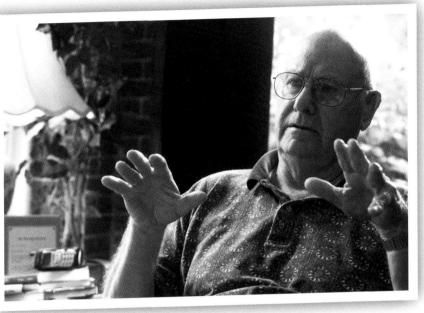

George Mann, founder and chairman of CORP, 1991-2012.

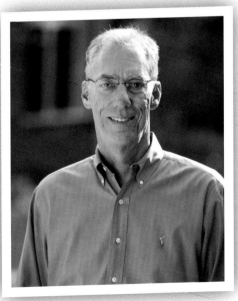

John Curtiss, Retreat co-founder
and president.

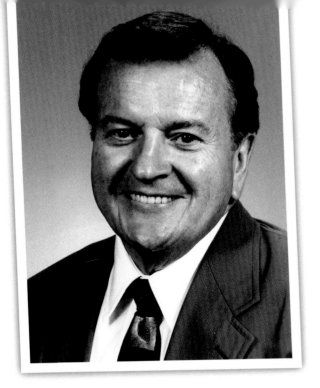

George Bloom, founding member of CORP
Board of Directors.

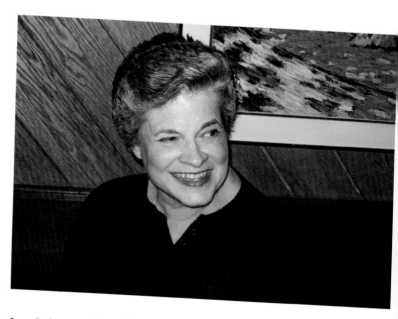

Jan Schwarz, founding member of CORP Board of Directors.

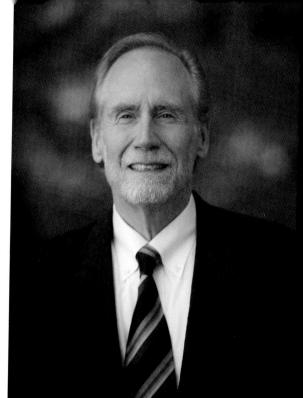

Terry Troy, chairman of CORP Board, 2012 to present.

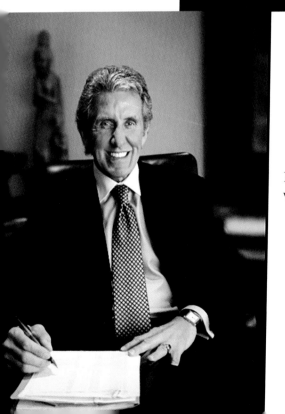

Dr. Peter Vogt, vice chairman

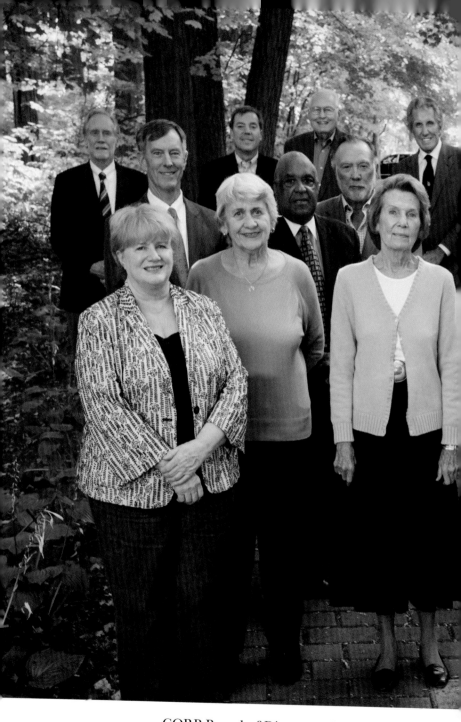

CORP Board of Directors, 2012.

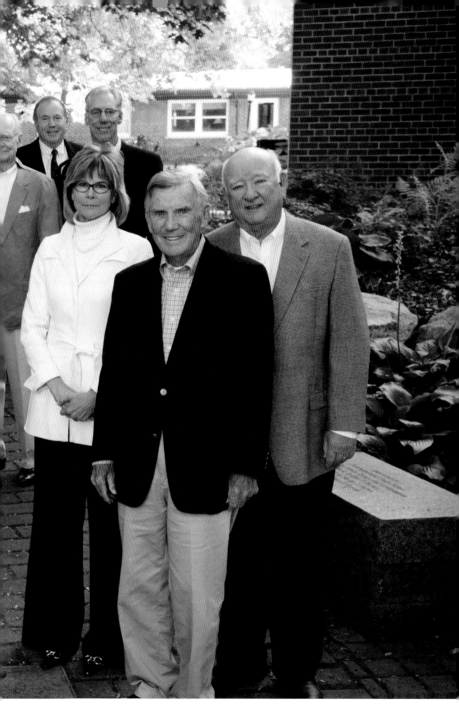

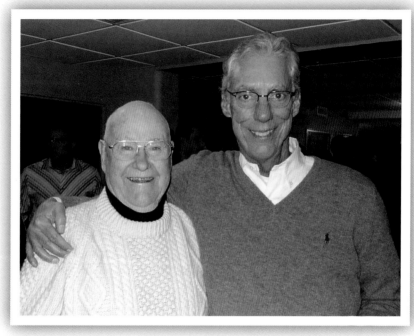

John and George at the 2010 Holiday Call-up meeting.

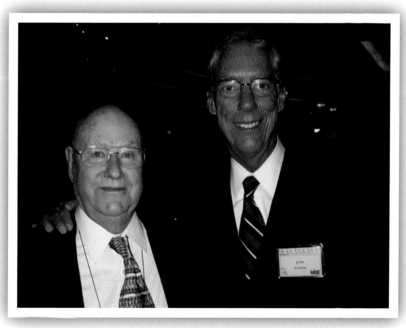

George and John at the Imagine event.

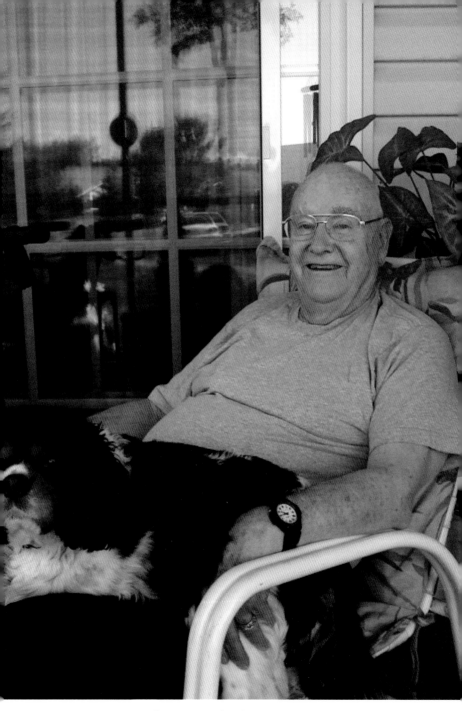

George and Winston.

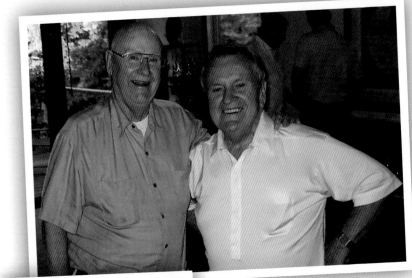

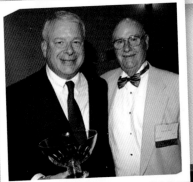

George Mann and
George Bloom.

Bob Bisanz receives
"Spirit of Community
Award" from George.

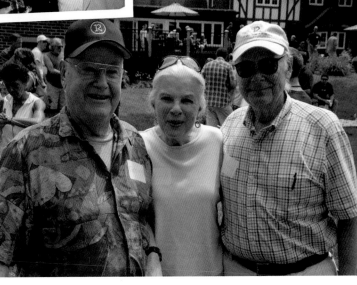

George Mann and Bob and Mary Harvey at the summer pic

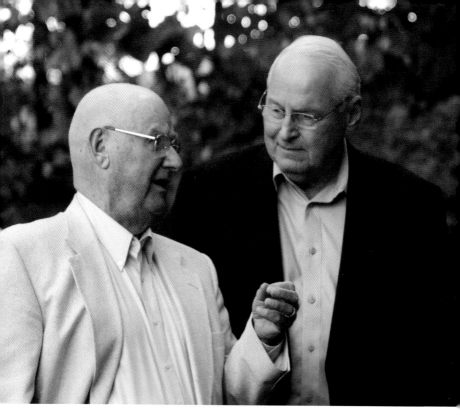

George Mann and Larry Koll.

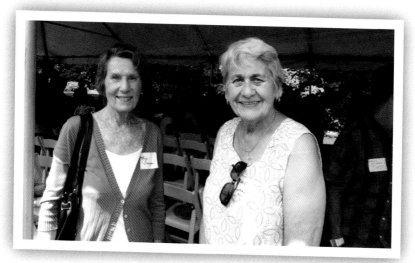

Gale Sharpe and Marie Manthey at the summer picnic.

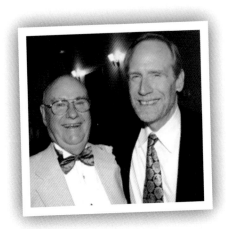

George Mann
and Terry Troy.

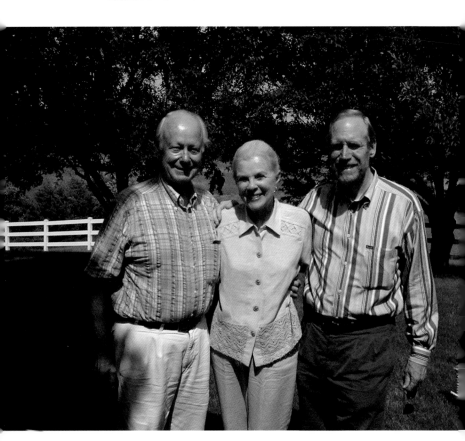

Bob and Mary Harvey and Terry Troy.

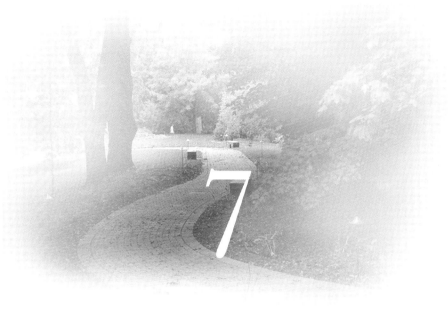

The Cenacle

Those early months and years at Upland Farms were inspirational. The board, the staff, and the hundreds of volunteers believed they were on to something unique and personally rewarding. Things came together to create a new mutual-help model of recovery. The staff, led by John Curtiss (whose vision and endurance counted for everything) and Diane Poole (who viewed recovery as a gift, not a burden), believed that Alcoholics Anonymous (AA) was all about love and service, in imitation of Dr. Bob. Recovery was to be found in the heart and not in the head. Curtiss and Poole had to support one another in those early days when they wondered and worried what the next challenge would be and when it would occur. There were, on occasion, issues around detox and physical and mental health, and it was not unusual for either of them, in the company of one or two other guests, to drive a guest to a clinic or hospital and sit there for hours.

Poole cherished Curtiss's role as both a good model and teacher, while he cherished her vision of loving people into recovery. He reminded Diane and the others that they were all in this together and could lean on one another for support. When they became anxious about how things were developing and the appearance of real or imagined road blocks, Curtiss would remind everyone that if it is meant to be, it will be.

Very early on, it became apparent that many of the guests needed more recovery time after finishing The Retreat program, some sort of sober housing—an option with which Curtiss had lots of personal and professional experience. He had gone through Hazelden's Fellowship Club as a resident, then served as its executive director, and eventually became president of the Association of Halfway House Alcoholism Programs of North America. The Retreat opened its first residence, a sober house, on Summit Avenue in the historic Crocus Hill area of St. Paul in 2000.

The whole idea was to allow the guests who graduated from The Retreat to become fully integrated into the recovering community in St. Paul. Settling into the residences provided them with the time, structure, and support essential to building a strong foundation for recovery. In the beginning, the cost was minimal—four hundred dollars a month.

The expectations were simple and manageable for those beginning recovery: both the men and the women had to find employment, work closely with a sponsor, attend a minimum of four AA meetings a week, and fulfill a weekly service commitment. Staff and volunteers met regularly with the residents to support their recovery and conduct *Alcoholics Anonymous: Big Book* studies.

At The Retreat at Upland Farms (Upland Farms was eventually dropped from the title), things gradually came together through the concerted efforts of the whole community and the personal energies and talents of the board, staff, and volunteers. Together, they created a sanctuary, a place of rest in which healing was evoked through the recovering circle of all those who came to carry the message and to practice these principles in all their affairs. Problems were addressed as they arose, and nothing was so big it couldn't be solved.

It wasn't long before the staff and directors realized that the major restriction on what they were accomplishing was that the manor was too small to accommodate all those seeking help. Not only were Sundays overflowing with families, guests, and pets, but also the number of beds limited those seeking admission. The solution was either to expand on the present site or seek another property that could accommodate more guests.

In 2001, three years after the opening of The Retreat, negotiations commenced for a piece of property on Game Farm Road, in Minnetrista, not far from Upland Farms. But these were put on hold and then ended when it was discovered that most of the neighbors opposed it, causing the City Planning Commission to veto it. It floundered principally on the issue of whether criminal background checks were being conducted on those admitted to The Retreat. (This was only a slightly different version of the public's attitude and perceptions of decades previous when alcoholics had been perceived as skid-row dwellers. Minnetrista was not the location for the new Retreat location.) Subsequent developments in cultivating good relationships with the Wayzata community took away the sting of rejection that recovering people had long come to expect. It was simply a matter of turning the other cheek and shaking the dust from their sandals.

But a crucial lesson had been learned. The board and the president of The Retreat realized that creating good relationships with the neighbors and city officials was crucial to establishing a facility in any new area. A site in downtown Wayzata became available in January 2003. It was called the Cenacle, a former retreat facility, located in the center of a strand of Minnesota's remaining Big Woods.

It came at an opportune time. The directors discovered that their mutual-help model worked and had come of age. The model had been tested and was not found wanting. In particular, the focus on helping the guests had shifted from a problem-based therapeutic model to one emphasizing solutions and relationships. Referrers were no longer skeptical or hesitant about sending people to The Retreat. There was an urgent need for more room and an imminent need for renovations. There was something of a meaningful synchronicity, or providence, between the need and the opportunity to purchase the Cenacle. A few of the directors of CORP had already remarked how the buildings and property would make a good fit for The Retreat's growing needs.

What was to become The Retreat's new home in Wayzata had a long history as a place for spiritual renewal and recovery. Centuries ago, the region's Dakota Indians regarded the land as holy because of its dense forests and nearby hills overlooking Lake Minnetonka. Later, European settlers revered it as part of the larger deciduous forest they called the Big Woods, a 6,500-square-mile area in Minnesota stretching north to St. Cloud and south to Mankato, and east to west from Northfield to the Minnesota River. In 2011, however, the Minnesota Department of Natural Resources estimated that only a small fraction of 1 percent of the original Big Woods was still standing.

The twenty-two-acre remnant in Wayzata is one part of that fraction, a small, dense forest of maple, oak, and basswood trees, some as much as 120 years old. The Big

Woods is a living system of diverse plant and animal life, and its deer-tracked trails are seasonally graced by jack-in-the-pulpits, bloodroot, anemone, cinnamon ferns, violets, early meadow rue, and pagoda dogwood shrubs.

In 1934, this parcel of the Big Woods was owned by Charles Sr. and Ruth Arnao, who that year built a large Tudor-style house on the property and named it the Greenridge Estate. The gracefully designed home formed the core of the main Cenacle retreat center, with six bedrooms, four bathrooms, four fireplaces, and a two-story living room.

Twenty-two years later, in 1956, the Arnao family sold the estate to the Sisters of the Cenacle, a Catholic order of nuns, who transformed the house into a retreat center, adding a chapel, two wings of sleeping rooms, and fourteen stations of the cross in the woods. The sisters changed the property's name to The Cenacle, which in the Bible refers to the upper room where Jesus and the disciples held the Last Supper. Later, the sisters sold the building to the first in a series of new owners with various plans—a private school and then an apartment and townhouse complex. These projects were dropped due to the fierce opposition of the citizens of Wayzata led by Merrily Borg Babcock, who formed The Friends of the Big Woods. They felt the development of the Big Woods would significantly increase both density and street traffic, eliminating the beautiful tree-lined view and posing a serious threat to Wayzata's small-town character and quality of life. To save the property from future development, The Friends of the Big Woods needed either to buy it or to find another buyer with a shared interest in preserving the Big Woods as well as the historic buildings.

For some time, The Retreat had needed more room to grow. Thanks to its advancing reputation as a successful and accessible model, its residential program at Upland Farms had an ever-increasing waiting list. Recognizing how the Cenacle could contribute to its growth, The Retreat joined forces with The Friends of the Big Woods, the Trust for Public Land and the City and Citizens of Wayzata. It was a unique partnership that was able to save the Big Woods through dedicated advocacy and fund raising.

The Retreat financed the $2 million purchase of the Cenacle building and just over seven acres of the land, while the other partners provided almost $4.9 million to purchase the remaining acres and preserve them in perpetuity. The Friends did this, with the assistance of The Retreat, by winning taxpayer support of a $3.1 million bond referendum that passed in November 2003, but not without a lot of hard work on the part of dedicated people to convince the citizens of Wayzata. The Friends of the Big Woods did a 2,000-piece mailing and put out yard signs throughout Wayzata. Curtiss attended sixteen community meetings promoting the referendum in various people's homes. Other board members were equally busy. Terry Troy, Dick Bisanz, and Curtiss spent much time negotiating the legal implications and formulated the language that went into the final documents. At the time, Wayzata had about 4,000 residents and 2,670 voters. Voter turnout was greater than 50 percent and the measure was approved by a slim margin of 51 votes, 734 to 683.

The collective success was a good example of the power of partnerships, a lesson learned when The Retreat had sought to purchase the property in Minnetrista. In the case of the Big Woods, everyone involved acknowledged that the whole enterprise would not have succeeded without the collaboration of all of the partners, especially in calming fears some citizens had about a recovery center in the middle of their city.

In actuality, the history of The Retreat is full of stories like these—people, opportunities, and resources showing up, aided by the dedication and commitment of a core of supporters. Mann said: "Both John [Curtiss] and I have felt God has guided us through this whole process. Call it serendipity. Call it miracles. It never would have happened without our Higher Power." The same sentiment was expressed by Mary Bader, one of the leaders of The Friends of the Big Woods who believed that The Retreat was the perfect community for the Cenacle property: "It has a healing spiritual mission just as the building had a healing spiritual mission for over fifty years."

Just as relationships and interconnectedness are essential and apparent throughout The Retreat's program, it was also apparent in The Retreat's partnership with the Wayzata community. Curtiss was the one most grateful for the relationships that developed in the long process in purchasing the property and saving the Big Woods. He believed that the people of Wayzata had embraced The Retreat from the beginning: "We provided an important piece of what was needed to save the Big Woods, and in the process we made a lot of friends."

The Retreat now owned the Cenacle. It opened in August 2004 with thirty beds, a 50 percent increase of Upland Farms, with a future capacity of up to seventy beds for the residential program. The city's conditional-use permit allowed The Retreat to maintain seventy beds in the main building and ten others in the single-family house that was also part of the purchased land. The future plan was to renovate and prepare another section of the Cenacle with twenty beds for family and spiritual retreat programs, the one alternating with the other every other week. The separate house on the grounds was initially envisioned as an interim step between The Retreat and its sober residences, accommodating ten guests who desired additional time and support after completing The Retreat's residential program.

In addition to providing a larger facility, the new property had the advantage of bringing The Retreat closer to its primary pool of volunteers in the Twin Cities. It had always emphasized the need for a strong relationship between its guests and the recovery community. An extensive base of volunteers provided The Retreat guests with living examples of recovery as well as personal support. Their participation also helped keep the program affordable. During a typical month's stay, guests met over three hundred volunteers "alive with the spirit of recovery" (according to John Curtiss). The volunteers met with the guests, individually and in groups, led *Alcoholics Anonymous: Big Book* studies, served as sponsors, provided an important link between the residential experience and the fellowship, and were engaged in the program of AA on a daily and lifelong basis. In the new location, The Retreat would be more accessible to its volunteers, while retaining a natural and private setting in the Big Woods.

While the purchase cost was $2 million, it was estimated that the renovations would require another $700,000. It was time to call upon the talents of Bruce Binger, the vice president in charge of development who had been so successful in the Campaign of Fellowship Drive, which ended in 2001 and raised $1.7 million. He was asked if he could raise three times that amount, $6 million over three years. When the capital campaign Making Room for Recovery (under the persuasive and committed leadership of CORP board member Dr. Peter Vogt) ended in October 2007, it had raised $6.5 million.

With the Cenacle, The Retreat had inherited a beautiful, quiet, meditative environment. The location was ideal. The building was spacious and much of the interior was very attractive. Still, much of the inner space needed extensive repair and remodeling. Diane Poole felt that the place had so many limitations that it was hard to know where to start. Her immediate impression was that the building was dark, dismal, and dank with a lot of asbestos under the carpets. While John and some volunteers were tearing up the carpet to remove the asbestos, she remembered that he kept reminding her not to look back at "what has been" but rather to look at "what will be." The architects assured her and John that the building could be restored and with creative redesign to recapture much of its original charm and sense of retreat for which the sisters had originally intended it.

In August 2004, Debbie Johnson, The Retreat's business manager, joined John at the new facility to help manage the pre-move logistics, with the actual move of guests from Minnetrista planned for September. The nostalgia for the old retreat was replaced by the nooks and crannies of the new, with its library, chapel, and meditation room, and the immediate opportunity to replace twenty beds with forty. It operated at near capacity for the rest of the year. In another wing, twenty beds were set aside for the family program, which occurred every other week. When this wing was vacated and the family program took up residence in the new

McIver Center for Family and Spiritual Care building in 2007, it was renovated and redesigned to become the Center for Women's Recovery, which allowed the women to have their own space and a gender-specific program.

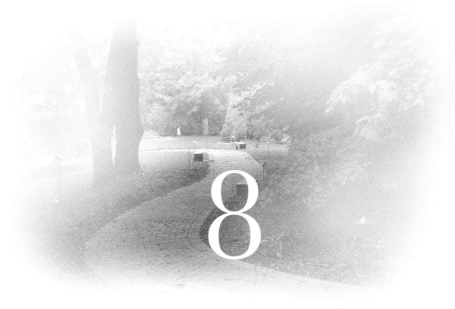

A Decade of Growth

Once comfortably ensconced in its new setting, The Retreat began to expand dramatically. Looking back from the vantage point of its tenth anniversary in 2007, The Retreat had grown from a concept of an affordable, spiritually grounded model of care to a $10 million organization that had helped thousands of alcohol- and drug-dependent individuals and families access recovery. At its heart, it remained a community that resisted institutionalization.

The Retreat had become a 134-bed continuum of recovery services that included a forty-bed men's center, a twenty-bed center for women's recovery, an eighteen-bed center for family and spiritual recovery, and a fifty-four bed long-term sober living program in four residences in the Crocus Hill area of St. Paul. Over three hundred volunteers came to The Retreat each month to carry a message of hope and recovery to the guests and their families. Their message was simple, focused, and from the heart about their personal recovery experiences. Every day, they modeled for the guests what it was like to be active and grateful members of the twelve-step recovery community.

The Retreat took pride in the numbers of people that it had assisted in the decade since it was first founded. It had served more than 5,500 individuals and families affected by alcoholism and drug dependency. By 2007, The Retreat's thirty-day program annually offered a healing sanctuary to 667 men and women, and its long-term sober-living residences had helped 106 people transition back into a meaningful life into the community. Since opening in 2005, the family program had served 525 family members and the center for spiritual development had helped over 900 individuals explore their spiritual journeys. The Retreat continued its commitment to ensure that people's inability to pay did not prevent them from receiving help by donating over $700,000 in making its services available to those who needed them.

In 2007, the programs for family and spiritual development had moved into the McIver Family Center, a beautiful new facility on the Wayzata campus. This allowed The Retreat to help hundreds of family members understand the effect of the disease of addiction on their lives and guide them into recovery. Family recovery is an essential component in long-term sobriety. The Retreat's program for families offered support, education, and hope to those most intimately affected by the disease of addiction. Family members frequently arrived bearing the confusion, pain, and despair so commonly caused by addiction. Three days later, most participants departed with hope and clarity. They understood more about the illness and its effects on them, they knew about actions they could take to improve their situation and support their loved ones, and they had learned about the role of spirituality in the deep healing necessary for recovery.

No space was left unused in the expansion of The Retreat's programs. The former space for the family program was converted into newly renovated living space for a retreat program designed specifically for women. The Retreat could now provide gender-specific recovery programs. Recognizing that alcoholism and drug dependency thrive in an atmosphere of isolation, building relationships among women was foundational to the women's program. Consequently, the program, led by Andrea Bruner, created a culture of trust and support where women could experience the power of recovery through community—both among resident guests and in fellowship with other female volunteers within the larger recovering community.

A vision of The Retreat's board from the beginning was to set in motion a national trend toward the development of more accessible and affordable recovery options for individuals and families needing help. As The Retreat evolved, demonstrated sustained growth, and maintained its stability, other groups showed interest in developing the same model in their communities. The Retreat offered to help replicate its own program for them by educating them in the value and practicality of the mutual help model of care. Up to this point, the field had been dominated by the professional treatment model.

The Recovering Community in Sioux Falls, South Dakota, was the first to successfully implement The Retreat's mutual help model. Relying on The Retreat for fund-raising methodologies, property design, and business procedures for running a residential program, the facility named Tall Grass opened in July 2006 with eighteen beds. The group, with the guidance of The Retreat, had already founded four sober houses with twenty-four beds, so now a solid continuum of services was in place. The success of The Retreat convinced the Tall Grass community that there was no question that what they were doing was the right thing.

In December 2008, the board formed a Replication Committee, which reported back in February of the following year that The Retreat was committed to two strategies: expansion and replication. Services had expanded in numerous ways over the past decade: sober housing, the family program, the women's program, evening programs, and the potential of a day program for seniors. By this time The Retreat had seen the replication of its model in Hong Kong and South Dakota and had provided assistance for many retreat-model sober houses throughout the country and abroad. However, the committee was also concerned about stretching leadership and finances at a time of uncertainty throughout the country. But keeping things in perspective, the board took pride that after a decade of growth, The Retreat was in a very solid financial condition.

"To remain an effective and credible organization requires constant vigilance, daily attention to the needs of our guests, and strict adherence to the mission. We strive to be a program of attraction, not of promotion. These constructs have guided our development from the beginning." With these thoughts, Bruce Binger, the vice president for development almost from the opening of The Retreat, summed up his own role in promoting its mission. His work had been nothing short of phenomenal. At the same time, he confessed that his job was made easier by the participants in the community of recovering people—guests, volunteers, board members, staff, and friends—all those who believe in its good purpose and wished to further the mission by contributing financially.

In 2007, the tenth anniversary of The Retreat marked the successful completion of a three-year fund-raising drive, Making Room for Recovery, which grossed $6.5 million. Started in the fall of 2004, the money raised was directed toward the purchase of the Cenacle property, the renovation of the facility, the establishment of the Guest Scholarship Fund, and the construction of the McIver Family Center. Combined with the previous Campaign of Fellowship fund-raiser, the grand total of $8 million was a remarkable sum and testimony to the wide support that The Retreat enjoyed over its first decade. It was able to provide over $700,000 in scholarships for nearly 800 men and women. (At the end of 2012, total donor giving had reached $14 million, of which 20 percent had come from the generosity of the board members.)

The seeds of a family program were planted early— in their original form in the month following the opening of The Retreat in Upland Farms in June 1998. After participating for three years at Upland Farms, Ellie Hyatt had moved on, but she was asked to come back as project coordinator for the Sunday afternoon meetings after The Retreat had moved into its new quarters at the Cenacle. Moreover, the time had arrived for the introduction of a family program. There were twenty extra beds that could be put to good use for a family program and spiritual retreats.

Both Curtiss and Mann had witnessed the great benefits and wisdom that families had absorbed from the family programs at St. Mary's and Hazelden, both based on the principles of Al-Anon and encapsulated in the phrase "Letting Go, Letting God." Their approaches were similar. The one divergence was whether or not the guest should be involved in the program at the same time that the family was present. The final decision was not to involve the guest with the immediate family. Curtiss and Mann came together to create a balanced approach to educate families about the character and consequences of chemical dependency and how they can care for themselves throughout the whole spiral of addiction and recovery.

In May 2005, Ellie was offered the position of director of the family program and urged to start one as soon as possible. She offered a program in July 2005, but only a few people signed up. In August, however, she was encouraged by the attendance of thirteen people. It was a marketing nightmare. She did her own in-house research, while consulting with other treatment centers. She found little enthusiasm and motivation among the guests for recommending it and a reluctance on the part of the staff to push it. The solution came in convincing the board to include the cost for one family member in the cost of care for the guest. This had a great effect on the attendance at the family program as enrollment doubled.

The construction of an eighteen-bed family center began in 2006 and it opened in the spring of 2007. The McIver Family Center (named after a grateful family who had pledged a significant donation) greatly enhanced and complemented Ellie's marketing efforts.

Initially, Ellie had nightmares about the program being removed from the Cenacle's main quarters because the program guests would have to walk through the snow in the winter and the mud in the spring to get to the Cenacle for certain exercises and meetings with the guests in the main building. However, a beautiful meandering path, built by a grateful alumni and his father, later connected the family center with the main buildings. The center's eighteen beds served the family program every other week. On the remaining weekends, it served as the Center for Spiritual Development, also under Ellie's direction, responding to a wide variety of audiences, some of whom found Dick Rice as their director.

The Retreat approach to the family program was educational and supportive. The participants found mutual support in the communal sharing with others. No one was alone on the recovery journey. Days spent at the center were meant to be a time of healing, not confrontation. A clear supposition was that the participants were doing the best that they could with the experience and knowledge that they had. The mutual sharing and the opportunity to identify with the experiences of others produced healing, just as Bill W. and Dr. Bob experienced in 1935.

The participants learned that they were not sick and needed neither doctor nor psychologist. By learning about the first three steps, they were introduced to the problem of powerlessness and the solution that could be found in a power greater than themselves. The solution was a spiritual one. The family program made reference to the beautiful words of the Jesuit anthropologist Pierre Teilhard de Chardin: "We are not human beings having a spiritual experience, but spiritual beings having a human experience."

The McIver Center, completed in 2007, was a sanctuary in which safe circles were created so that the participants could speak from their hearts—*cor ad cor loquitur*, that is "one heart speaking to another." The guests learned about meditation and prayer, and about the value of the practice of their personal stories, which hopefully would become habitual when the guests left the program. The knowledge they received was the same knowledge given to the recovering guests in the residential program. They discovered that telling their stories to other human beings was sacred ground.

Original Staff

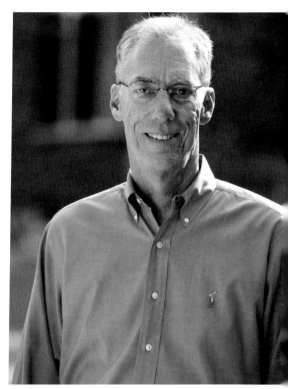

John Curtiss,
president and
employee number one.

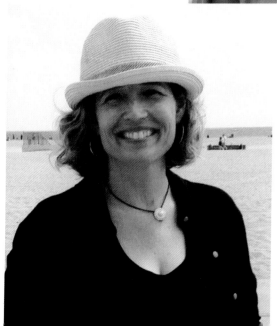

Misha Quill,
employee number
two, The Retreat's
first admissions
coordinator.

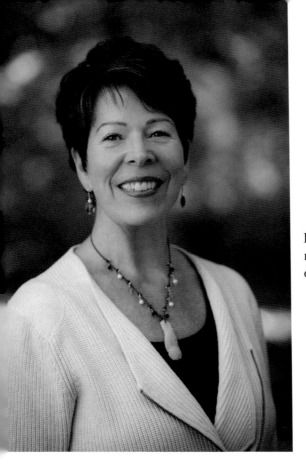

Diane Poole, employee number three, program director

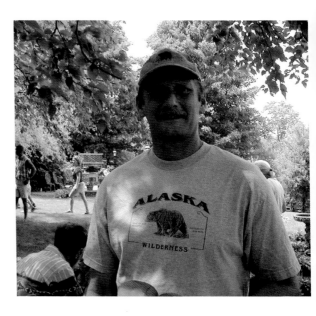

Greg Olson, employee number four, overnight Retreat assistant.

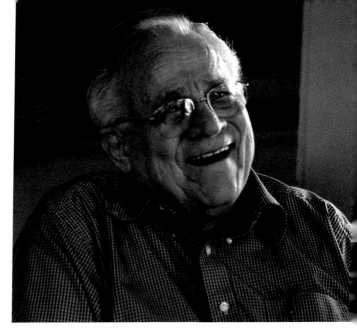

Duane Jackson "DJ," spiritual director,
1998-2012.

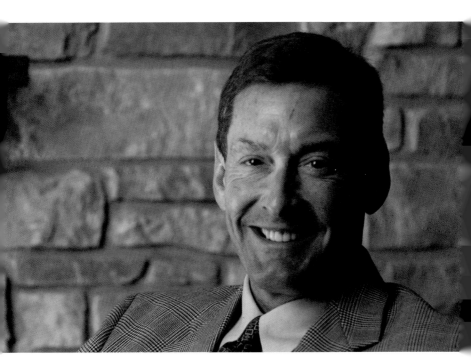

Retreat Vice President of Development Bruce Binger,
1998-2013.

Staff & Volunteers

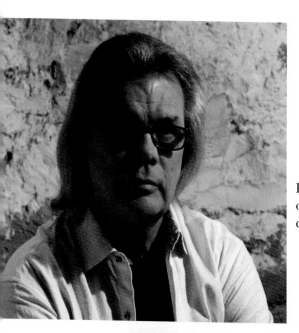

Roger Bruner, designer of Retreat's *Big Book* study curriculum.

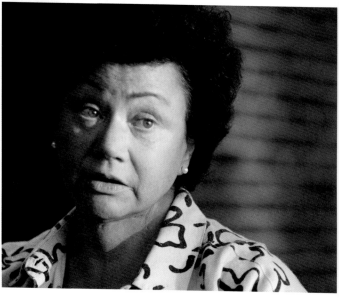

Cookie S., *Big Book* instructor.

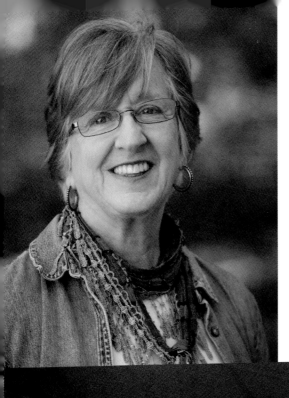

Ellie Hyatt,
family volunteer
coordinator.

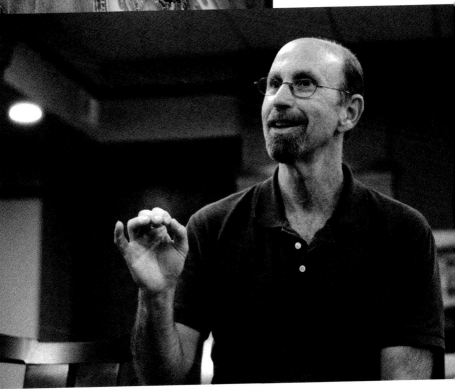

Marc Hertz (Meditation Marc).

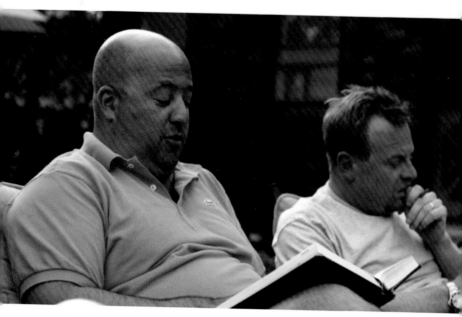

Andrew Z. and Aaron M., Residence *Big Book* volunteers.

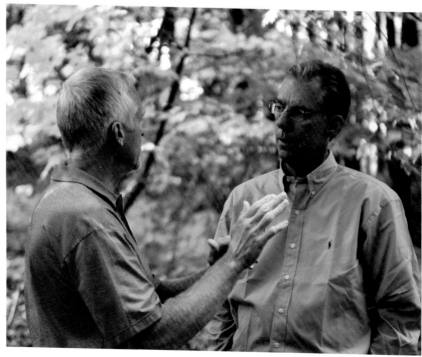

Jack Odom (Men's Program Coordinator) and John Curtiss.

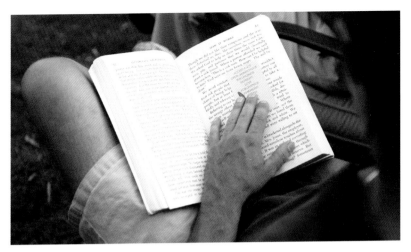

Alcoholics Anonymous Big Book, the primary curriculum of The Retreat.

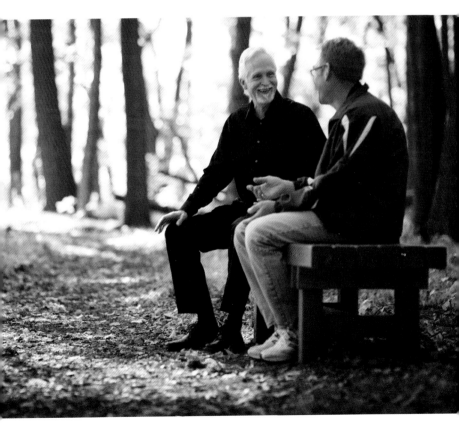

Jack Odom and Bill Oliver.

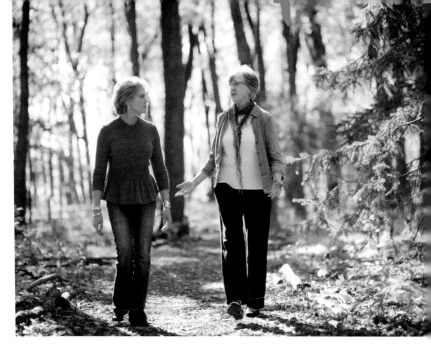
Debbie Jones and Ellie Hyatt.

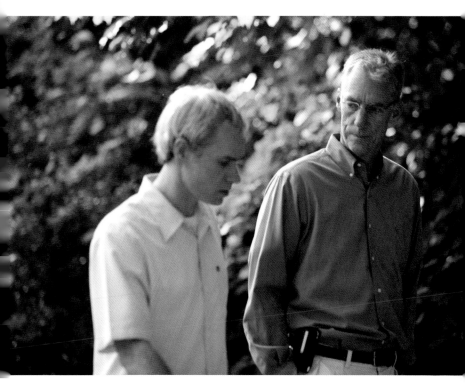
John Leonard and John Curtiss.

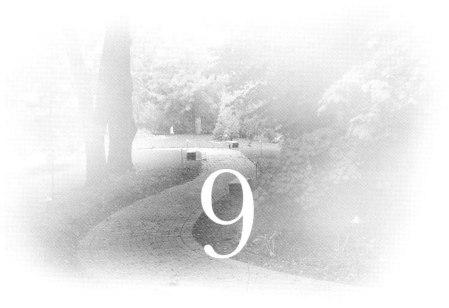

9

The Challenge of Growth

The Retreat's president, John Curtiss, was very much aware of the challenges the organization encountered as it moved into its new building and enlarged its circle of services. Undertaking the renovation of the new facility, planning for new and expanded services, and kicking off a fund-raising campaign to support this growth all contributed to a certain unease that the growth might be too much and too fast, resulting in the loss of intimacy that wrapped itself around the smallness (humility) of The Retreat at Upland Farms.

Curtiss faced the challenge head on. How does one grow and stay small? He wrote: "Not unlike the residents of Wayzata, who have supported the purchase of the Big Woods to preserve the intimacy and character of their own community, we at The Retreat are committed to preserving the quality of our community and program in these next stages of growth." He recognized the need for The Retreat and those closely connected with it—staff, volunteers, and board members—to go slowly and to pay attention to all the elements of the program and not just to add for the sake of adding.

Curtiss continued: "Certainly, we will need to expand our staff and increase our budget. But we will not fill the new building all at once. Rather, we will grow into it over time, ever conscious that recovery requires space. We will remain focused on fostering and preserving the intimate community setting, the personal relationships, and the spiritual focus that have been our priority from the beginning and will continue to be the hallmark of our success."

On the occasion of The Retreat's tenth anniversary, it was time to take stock, to do an inventory. "A business which takes no regular inventory usually goes broke. . . . It is a fact finding and fact facing process. . . . One object is to disclose damaged or unsalable goods, to get rid of them promptly and without regret. If the owner of the business is to be successful, he cannot fool himself about values" (*Alcoholics Anonymous*, 64).

In December 2008, the Board of Directors held its own retreat to look back upon the accomplishments of the previous decade. It was an opportunity to recognize how much they had accomplished with a small, dedicated staff. Curtiss presented an impressive list of accomplishments since The Retreat's opening.

Growing from 19 to 134 beds and from 4 to 44 employees allowed The Retreat to reach out to some 6,400 people. As a result of Curtiss's strong management skills and the strong financial background of The Retreat's director of business operations, Debbie Johnson, the business side was running efficiently and annually in the black. What was most important was that The Retreat had gained an excellent reputation in the Alcoholics Anonymous (AA) and professional communities. It had raised $9.5 million with the support of over 1,800 donors. The Annual Imagine Galas and Golf Extravaganzas had become phenomenal successes. Over $170,000 in scholarships were distributed in 2008, 8.5 percent of the total revenue for the year. (Time and history do not stand still. As this volume goes to press in February 2014, The Retreat has served over 15,000 guests since it opened and has raised over $15 million from 3,800 donors. The financial support for scholarship funds has increased from $1.6 million in 2008 to $2.5 million in 2013.) The Retreat's sober-house model had been replicated in many communities, nationally and internationally. The family program and the spiritual retreat center program had helped hundreds, and a new nonresidential evening program had been established in Wayzata, which was soon to be followed by one in St. Paul. The outpatient program evolved from a discussion with several the business community, who had expressed an interest in such a program. In the corporate world, more businesses were sending their employees to outpatient programs. The evening program, like the residential program, sober residences, and soon-to-be-created online recovery programs all represented The Retreat's commitment to creating new, accessible, and affordable recovery models.

It was made clear at the outset that The Retreat's nonresidential programs, however, would not be based on a treatment model, but would be educational and supportive, similar to its residential model already in place. It had two components: The Evening Essential (primary program) and The Evening Enrichment (continuing care). AA meetings were part of the program, not optional. Guests were encouraged to create sustaining relationships with sober individuals. This outpatient initiative was seen as completing The Retreat's circle of services.

Curtiss felt that the Evening Program might be the best model to replicate as a way to establish a presence in a community without being overly burdened with capital-intensive brick-and-mortar projects. New York, Chicago, Dallas, and Seattle appeared to be good locations for a trial run beyond the friendly confines of the Twin Cities. The big question was how to integrate the existing recovering community and the volunteer members that come from within it, an essential element of The Retreat methodology of recovery.

The same question applied as The Retreat pursued the possibility of another unique program—myRecovery.com. In an effort to help more people recover and bring the vast resources of recovery-related information together into one easily accessible format, The Retreat began to develop myRecovery.com. An online recovery resource would offer three key components: a social networking site designed specifically for people in recovery, an online recovery program using video-conferencing technology to bring people together face-to-face to support each other in their first few months of recovery, and a comprehensive resource directory of recovery-related information. It did not seem difficult to create modules for screening, recovery principles, family, and continuing care with social networking and video conferencing interwoven with each module. But the bigger question was: Would this service be able to create the kind of mutual sharing community so essential to The Retreat model?

As The Retreat moved into the second decade of its mission to help as many people as possible, the unique model it had created and was sharing had grown beyond the imaginations of the original founders. Some of those founders had begun to wonder at what point The Retreat might begin to lose its personal touch and its spirit of smallness. "Robert Harvey was one such board member who continually reminded us to keep our eye on our original mission," Curtiss recalled.

Smallness was not necessarily a quantitative issue but a qualitative attitude that was given its best expression in the seventh step with the use of the word *humbly*. Humility has a variety of meanings. One important meaning comes from the recognition that there is someone higher and more powerful—a higher power upon which we are dependent and that stands in stark contrast with our self-centeredness. And indeed, it is to this higher power that The Retreat owes its success—a recognition that God could do for us what we could not do for ourselves. This was evident every step of the way in the story of The Retreat:

Allowing the mission to unfold through the
path of mutual help.

Finding the key recovering people to
implement the project.

Acquiring the first beautiful facility
and environment.

Following the road less traveled to the Cenacle.

The generosity of The Retreat's supporters.

An ever-broadening continuum of services.

Inspired leadership.

Indeed, all things had come together for good. No need to worry about too much growth if the community could remain humble and teachable.

This required that The Retreat maintain its philosophy of mutual help, the importance of the community, the recognition that it was not one but many walking the road of happy destiny, the belief that there was a power greater than self at work here, and the certainty that what counted were relationships and not rugged individualists in the grand scheme of things.

To maintain the personal touch, the following were needed: (1) the practice of both personal and professional inventories to prevent The Retreat from becoming an institution and losing the community ideal; (2) an inventory that would permit The Retreat to keep the balance between continuity, change, and growth; (3) an ongoing commitment and dedication of the board, staff, and volunteer community to grow in their own recovery programs and anchor themselves in the spirituality of the program and the kit of spiritual tools essential to sobriety and sanity.

Still, there was much to be done. Between 1990 and 2000, the United States had surrendered 60 percent of its residential treatment beds. Most disturbing was that Minnesota, once the gold standard of treatment in the world, was ranked forty-eighth among the fifty states in the ability to access treatment since costs for residential care could amount to 50 percent of a family's income. Residential stays were reduced to three to six days. Some believe that any residential treatment less than fourteen days was hardly worth the effort.

Since 1990, driven by medical-necessity criteria, there had been a much greater emphasis on assessing and treating co-occurring mental health issues. CORP acknowledged that some, with more serious mental health conditions could, and should, be treated early in the treatment process. However, many of the issues identified in the first few weeks of sobriety would likely disappear with total abstinence from mood-altering chemicals, active involvement in Alcoholics Anonymous and the gift of time—or could just as easily be treated in a continuing care environment. There was a diminishing focus on teaching the Twelve Step principles of recovery and the spiritual healing disciplines that underlay them. As chemical dependency moved under the umbrella of behavioral health and psychiatry, a greater emphasis was placed on biochemical interventions to address the problem.

It was against this backdrop that The Retreat was doing its own intervention by holding up a mirror to the field and reflecting in it the problem and the simplicity of the solution.

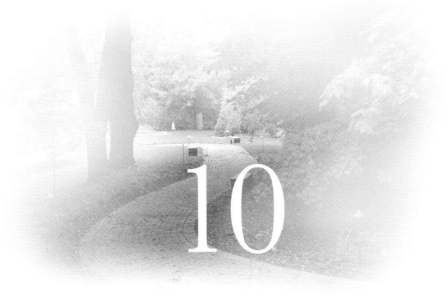

10

The Practice of These Principles

"Women Suffer Too," one of the stories in the *Alcoholics Anonymous: Big Book*, contains a striking passage that helps highlight the spiritual nature of recovery. The author writes: "I went trembling into a house in Brooklyn filled with strangers . . . and I found that I had come home, at last, to my own kind. There is another meaning for the Hebrew word that in the King James' version of the Bible is translated 'Salvation.' It is 'to come home.' I had found my salvation—I wasn't alone anymore."

Dr. Bob's walk in recovery began in his relationship with another drunk. He was no longer alone. That conversation provided the stage for an individual's recovery. It was also the spiritual foundation of the recovery movement.

"One description of addiction is that it is a

pathological relationship of love and trust with alcohol or drugs in place of relationships with our real selves, with others, and with the God of our understanding" (*The Addictive Personality*, 10–11). In this sense, recovery is relinquishing our connection with chemicals and rediscovering and recovering our natural threefold relationship.

The program of The Retreat can be reduced to a simple spiritual protocol: Participation in the fellowship/community of Alcoholics Anonymous (AA) and the practice of the principles of the Twelve Steps in all of our affairs. The fellowship that emerged in 1935 was the first element of the recovery protocol. The second element was the kit of spiritual tools revised and accepted by the growing fellowship and found in the *Alcoholics Anonymous: Big Book* completed in 1939.

The ritual of walking through the doors of The Retreat, of coming home, introduces a person to a community of people, from every shire's end, who have the same or similar problems and have arrived at a crossroads in their journeys. They can either continue on the same path, blotting out the consciousness of their intolerable situation or accept spiritual help (*Alcoholics Anonymous*, 25). Of course, crossing the threshold of The Retreat, they were unaware of exactly what they were doing except that they needed to change.

After being introduced to the ordinary routine of the day, like eating, sleeping, and wondering what will be expected of them, they are further put at ease as the other guests of The Retreat talk, listen, and share their stories with them. As the days progress, they learn that these simple human practices will be essential to their recovery. They discover that in these simple conversations there is a remarkable similarity of experiences. It is through this mutually shared vulnerability that one will find the solution.

From the start, another group of strangers make an appearance. These are the recovering men and women anxious to tell the guests about their own personal lives—what happened to them and what life is like for them now in contrast to what it was like before. All of them offer hope and friendship, and some of them become their teachers by including them in the circle of recovering people and providing the insights into the treasures of *Alcoholics Anonymous: Big Book*. They explain that the purpose of the book is to help those who read it find a Higher Power: "Lack of power, that was our dilemma. We had to find a Power by which we could live, and it had to be a Power greater than ourselves. Obviously. But where and how were we to find this Power? Well, that's exactly what this book is about. Its main object is to enable you to find a Power greater than yourself which will solve your problem" (*Alcoholics Anonymous*, 45).

The new guests listened, a few going through the motions, but many more curious, asking questions and sharing their own experiences of their personal descent into hell. They begin to find strength in the community.

Belonging to this community was the cornerstone of a Higher Power through which the God of their understanding would speak to them about their chemical dependency.

As the recovering group of sharers took them past chapter 4 of the *Alcoholics Anonymous: Big Book*, the guests began to learn about the kit of spiritual principles—the Twelve Steps—that would become the tools to help them reconnect with themselves, others, and the God of their understanding. They were introduced to Bill W.'s *Twelve Steps and Twelve Traditions*, which was especially helpful in fleshing out the meaning of each step.

These recovering men and women teach the guests about the practices of personal inventory, prayer, and meditation and the need to carry the message to others to safeguard and strengthen their own recovery. The third, fourth, and tenth steps receive special attention, with a tenth-step group every evening that continues to take personal inventory. The guests are expected to do an in-depth study of steps one through eight. Seeking out a sponsor from the volunteers lays the groundwork for a relationship that is crucial to recovery and to spiritual growth.

Gradually, the minds of most of the guests are opened and the clarity of their powerlessness becomes evident to them. They now have the knowledge and determination to remain sober. But knowledge and willpower can be deceptive tools and terribly misleading: "Above all he believed he had acquired such a profound knowledge of the inner working of his mind and its springs that relapse was unthinkable. Nevertheless he was drunk in a short time" (*Alcoholics Anonymous*, 26). Many of the guests at The Retreat have already been residents there and elsewhere and had failed. One had to go far beyond self-knowledge and willpower.

A recurrent theme of the *Alcoholics Anonymous: Big Book* is that self-knowledge, including knowledge of one's illness, does not provide the alcoholic with an adequate defense against the first drink (the merciless obsession).

For those who really wanted recovery, they discovered that the *Alcoholics Anonymous: Big Book* is not simply recommending a Higher Power relationship to free oneself from alcohol and drugs. It is also advancing the idea that the alcoholic's basic problem is his/her self-sufficient ways—ways that have closed the channel to the higher power. The alcoholic must rid himself of the self-centeredness through steps three and eleven and embrace the humility that speaks to something bigger than the self. For those who hide behind their agnosticism or their inability to accept a God of their understanding, *Twelve Steps and Twelve Traditions* is more than clear that the group is a more than adequate replacement for one's Higher Power.

The personal stories in the *Alcoholics Anonymous: Big Book* are the legacy of those who believe in the recovery journey and are there for inspiration and imitation. But it is the active community and fellowship of recovering alcoholics that hold the essential key to a life of sobriety.

Consequently, AA meetings are central to an individual's path to sobriety.

There can be no mistake: living the principles and participation in the fellowship to which the AA participants in The Retreat give testimony are the heart and soul of AA spirituality. Recovery is possible for all participants if they are willing to go to any lengths.

The spirituality of the program started with the significant insight of Bill W. and Dr. Bob, who in conversations with one another came to the special insight that recovery can take place with one alcoholic sharing his story with another alcoholic.

This insight into mutual sharing is no better illustrated than in the essay in *Alcoholics Anonymous: The Big Book* titled "Dr. Bob's Nightmare":

[Bill W.] gave me information about the subject of alcoholism which was undoubtedly helpful. *Of far more importance was the fact that he was the first living human with whom I had talked, who knew what he was talking about from actual experience. In other words he talked my language.* He knew all the answers, and certainly not because he had picked them up in his reading. (*Alcoholics Anonymous*, 180, emphasis added)

This was the foundation for mutual help and from that point forward the great gift that one alcoholic could give to another was his/her own personal experiences— well digested. No one can say there is nothing spiritual going on in their lives. Telling your story to another human being is sacred ground.

Current Staff

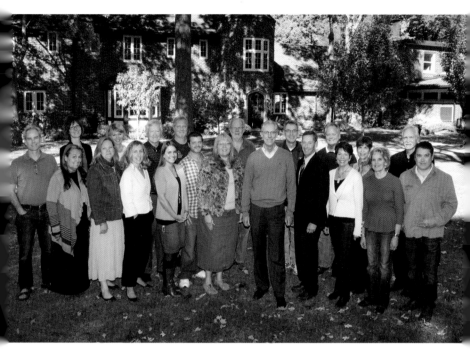

Retreat Staff 2012 — Into action!

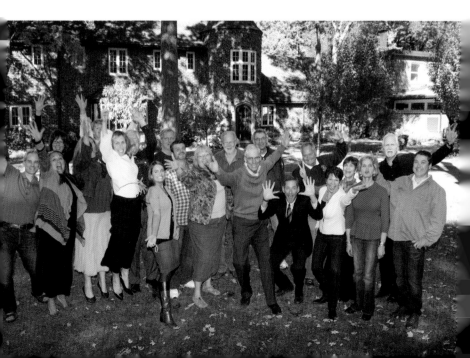

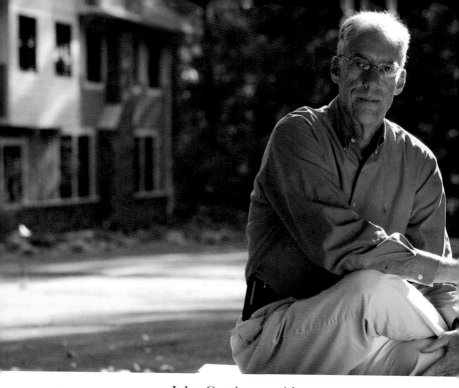

John Curtiss, president.

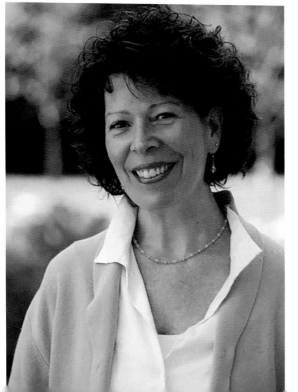

Diane Poole,
program director.

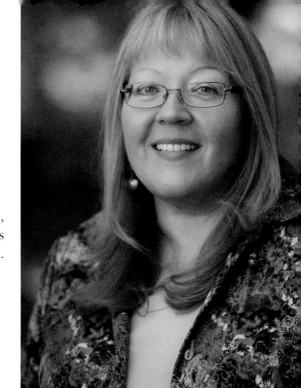

Debbie Johnson,
director of Business
Operations.

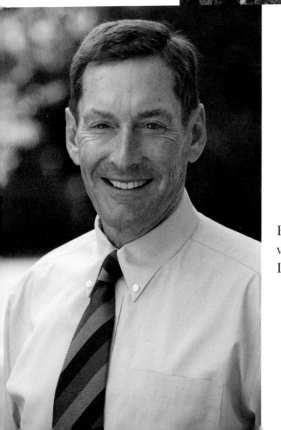

Bruce Binger,
vice president of
Development, 1998-2013.

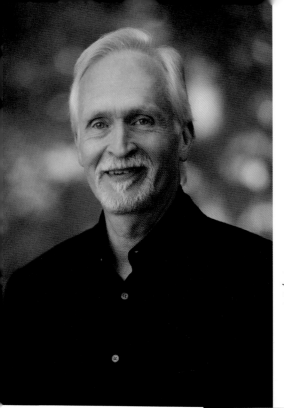

Jack Odom, men's
program coordinator

Andrea Bruner,
women's program
coordinator.

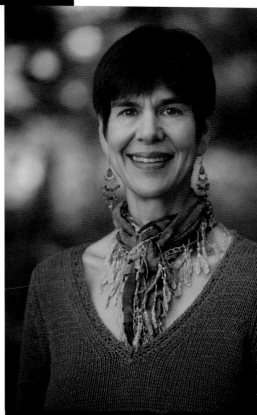

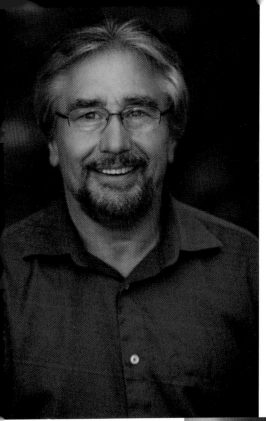

Mike Jamison, director
of Non-residential
Services.

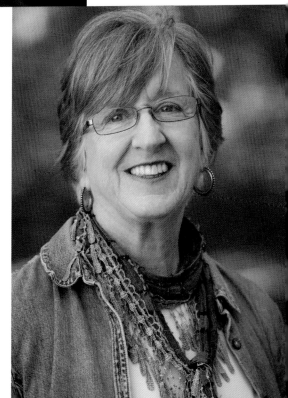

Ellie Hyatt, director
of Family and
Spiritual Care.

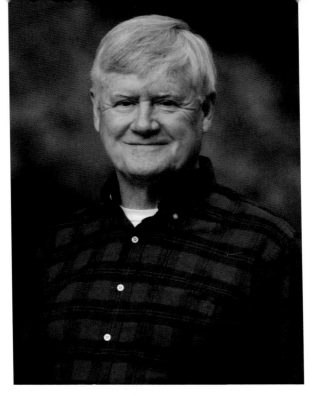

Dick Rice, director of Spiritual Care.

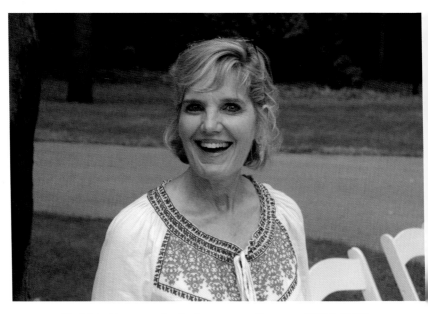

Debbie Jones, admissions coordinator, 2004-2013.

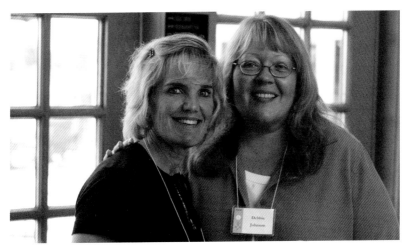

Debbie Jones and Debbie Johnson at our Golf Extravaganza.

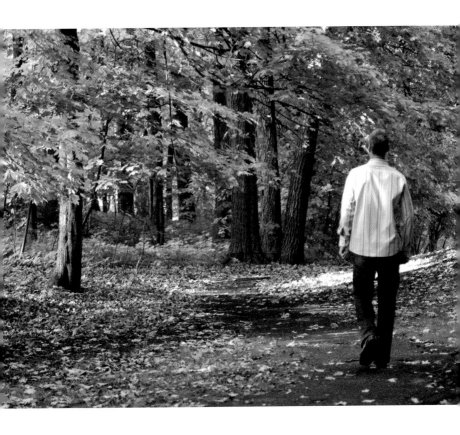

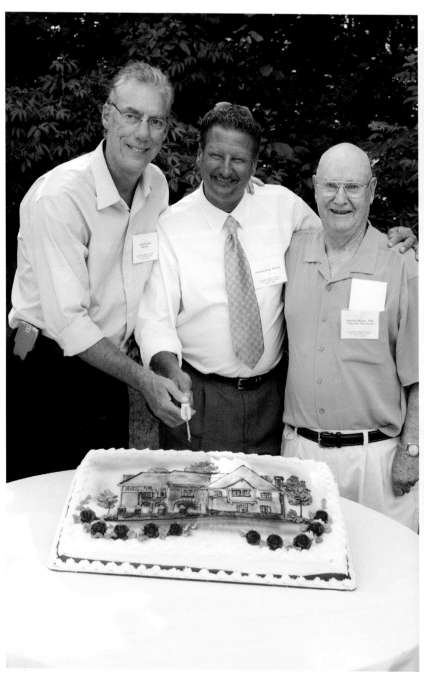

2007 opening of McIver Center for Family & Spiritual Recovery
with Christopher McIver cutting the cake.

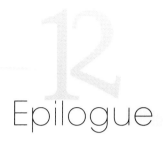

Epilogue

An Essay on the Minnesota Model

The story of The Retreat has a context that reveals how important, even revolutionary, the emergence of The Retreat was. The context is the evolution of the Minnesota model of treatment, an evolution from a model of mutual help to one of institutional and professional treatment. It also provides a classic example of the initial clash between the two and the reasons for that dialectic. It highlights the tension between community and institutionalism and the struggle between continuity and change to maintain what is essential while embracing the novel and the relevant.

What was attractive and significant about the Minnesota model at the pinnacle of its fame and influence was the dignity and respect that it rendered to each individual coming for its care, the importance of the value of community that it inspired, and the concentration on the Twelve Steps of Alcoholics Anonymous (AA) as elements of a lifelong recovery. All of these and others played into the education of John Curtiss at Hazelden and Dr. George Mann at St. Mary's Hospital.

Eventually, they both reacted strongly to the demands and directions of managed care and their interpretations of insurance coverage. At about the same time, they concluded that the rising cost of care, the excessive focus on co-occurring mental disorders, the multiplication of services, and the loss of a simple, direct approach to treatment based upon the Twelve Steps and spiritual principles of AA were complicating the Minnesota model. They were causing the loss of its simplicity and limiting its access to the many people who could benefit from participation in the program.

In the last analysis, the recovery path laid out by the Minnesota model in its earliest stages had been hijacked. Mutual help and the simple protocol of fellowship and steps became buried in the thicket of professionalism. Finally, most treatment centers could not adapt to the increased demands put upon them by the insurance companies and the new "more advanced" models of treatment.

It was in this context that The Retreat was born, recapturing the significant discovery of Bill W. and Dr. Bob, who in their conversations with one another came to the special insight that recovery can take place with one alcoholic talking to another. Describing their talk "as a completely mutual thing," Bill said: "I had quit preaching. I knew I needed this alcoholic as much as he needed me. *This was it*" (*Dr. Bob and the Good Old Timers*, 68, emphasis added). And this mutual give and take is at the very heart of all of AA's Twelve Step work today.

The fellowship that emerged in 1935 was the first element of the recovery protocol. The second was the kit of spiritual tools—the Twelve Steps—revised and accepted by the growing fellowship and found in *Alcoholics Anonymous: The Big Book* originally completed in 1939.

New York and Akron

Even before the publication of *Alcoholics Anonymous: The Big Book*, the protocol was being passed on in the meetings held in the Wilson home in New York City, and the Smith and Williams homes in Akron, Ohio—places where the squads experienced the primitive immersion in the developing practices and principles of AA. Those alcoholics who needed a place to stay found temporary sanctuaries in these homes. They became mutual-sharing circles as well the occasional place to rest for the penurious or sleep for the inebriated. In those early days, carrying the message was slow going and demanded great sacrifices. For Bill and his wife Lois, caring for this motley crew was a great hardship, for they too were short of funds.

Bill's early visions of paid missionaries and a number of hospitals throughout the United States for alcoholics remained dreams. However, they did come true in other forms. Dr. Bob, along with Sister Ignatia, was able to establish a ward in St. Thomas Hospital in Akron where alcoholics could be detoxed and, with the mutual help of AA members from the community, be initiated and immersed in the program and practice of AA.

St. Thomas Hospital and High Watch Farm

In the St. Thomas program, the hospital provided the necessary medical detoxification while an AA sponsor of the patient was in charge of his education about the program, which extended over five days. The sponsor and the senior patients provided the welcome and encouragement the first day. On the second day, the patients were guided through the first three steps. Days three and four were given over to a moral inventory and letting go of the past. On day five, the sponsor and patient discussed the patient's aftercare—his plans for the future—and living outside of the hospital and practicing the principles of AA in all his affairs.

Contemporaneously, the seminal idea of professional treatment found its expression in High Watch Farms in Kent, Connecticut. There, besides offering a place for guests to reflect on their recovery and the AA program, they were also afforded the opportunity to attend classes on a variety of topics offered by a recovering lay psychologist. Marty Mann was particularly incensed at seeing High Watch move in this direction. With the help of Bill W., High Watch returned to its original form and purpose of mutual help.

While the Minnesota model has a long history, we shall touch only briefly on those parts that illustrate its evolution from a mutual help model to one of professional treatment. This will provide the context for the development of The Retreat, which, given its history and location, might fittingly be labeled Minnesota model II.

Pat Cronin

The central figure in the AA movement in Minnesota was Pat Cronin. He spread the message as no one else did. He was tireless in bringing the good news of recovery not only to Minnesota, but also throughout the Midwest. Approximately 450 groups trace their establishment to his direct or indirect influence.

After a long history of alcohol abuse and then

dependence, he decided he needed to do something about his drinking but did not know where to turn to get help. In 1940, after reading a part of *Alcoholics Anonymous: The Big Book*, he wrote to the Alcoholic Foundation in New York City telling them that he had checked the book out of the public library, but he felt that he needed somebody to "lean on, if the book is right, who knows what I am up against." In other words, it takes an alcoholic to know an alcoholic, and he needed mutual help. On the tenth of November, two Chicago natives who had been attending a Minnesota–Michigan college football game barged in on him to give him the AA workout. The following day, the infamous Black Blizzard struck Minnesota, claiming many lives and bringing travel to a complete halt. Because the pair could not return to Chicago, they had some extra days "to work on Cronin." His dry date became November 11, 1940. From that point forward, it "was time to give what he had received." Cronin was indefatigable in spreading the good news of recovery, and his influence on the growth of AA throughout the Midwest was preeminent.

The Minneapolis Club

The year after his recovery, Pat Cronin and others founded the Minneapolis Club for the recovering community in Minneapolis. Known simply as the Club or 2218, it was a model for receiving, instructing, and nurturing those who had the simple and singular desire to stop drinking. In those early days, induction into AA came not through treatment but by AA immersion and mutual help. *Alcoholics Anonymous: The Big Book* contained the key to recovery, and its message was to be passed on through oral tradition. That was how it evolved at 2218.

As it grew, the group was divided into small units, called squads. In the very early days, it was taken for granted that potential AA members were not people accustomed to reading books. When someone arrived at 2218, not sure of what he was getting into, he was taken to Cronin with the request that he explain AA to the new person. From this evolved the discussion group or classes. In the beginning, Pat would explain the Twelve Steps to the new person in one class or discussion.

Not long after, the Twelve Steps were divided into four discussions or classes (similar to the model used at St. Thomas Hospital). The pattern for the Midwest was as follows: Class 1—Step 1; Class 2—Steps 4, 5, 8, and 9 (Inventory and Restitution); Class 3—Steps 2, 3, 6, 7, 10, and 11 (Spiritual); and Class 4—Step 12. Soon other groups added their own related materials, but the Twelve Steps were always the fundamental topics to be passed along in the community and fellowship of recovering alcoholics.

The tradition handed on to the novices, besides the written word, *Alcoholics Anonymous: The Big Book*, was the recovering alcoholic's personal understanding and experience of the steps, program, and process of AA taught through the older members' personal stories and examples. AA squads and meetings under the direct or indirect influence of Cronin multiplied rapidly throughout Minnesota.

Pioneer House

Besides his direct or indirect influence on the many AA groups established throughout the Midwest, Cronin founded Pioneer House, which was a retreat setting rather than a treatment setting on property offered by the Union City Mission on Medicine Lake. The bulk of the referrals came from AA, the welfare department, the municipal court system, and probation officers. Pat could regularly be found in court looking for men who might benefit from the program and convincing judges of the value of Pioneer House. In turn, the welfare department saw the potential benefits and the substantial cost savings of sobering up people whose families were a recurring burden on the city's relief roles.

Cronin developed a series of fifteen lectures on the Twelve Steps on "how recovery takes place and how the various phases of the program work." There were two formal meetings during the day: one on recovery topics and the other on the AA program. Small-group sessions and individual counseling were all part of the immersion. Pat believed that what alcoholics needed most was a feeling of acceptance by society, given their previous experience of total rejection.

There was a minimum of rules and regulations. The clients were given two books: *Alcoholics Anonymous: The Big* Book and the *Twelve Steps and Twelve Traditions.* They were expected to complete the first five steps before leaving treatment. The willingness to get honest was the essential element of recovery, and Pat was a strong believer in the use of the fourth and fifth steps, which were required of everyone. "Do it or stay [at Pioneer House] forever" was the working principle. The spiritual dimensions of recovery were emphasized from day one.

Cronin was known as the grand pappy of AA in the Midwest. He sponsored hundreds of recovering people. One of these was Lynn Carroll, founder and director of Hazelden, the Guest House established in 1949. In Cronin's twenty-four years of sobriety, he helped more than 30,000 people, and some 450 AA groups had his imprint. He lived the message and passed it on. In the midst of the many squabbles that recovering people could get into, he kept AA united and together. It is the mark of the man that his recovery came first and then the recovery of others.

Hazelden

Hazelden is the best example of a mutual-help model that evolved into one of professional treatment. Before it retained the original name of Hazelden, the intention had been to call it "Guest House." It was to be a haven of mutual help, but over the years morphed into a professional treatment center of world renown and the primary example of the Minnesota model. Its evolution provides a paradigm closely resembling the origins of The Retreat. Hazelden, which was founded the year after Pioneer House, was a retreat-like setting where mutual help was central to the recovery process. Lynn Carroll, a recovering alcoholic and a friend and disciple of Cronin, was keenly interested in the model that Cronin was developing at Pioneer House.

Hazelden (named after Hazel Power, formerly Hazel Thompson of the Thompson family, which owned the Pioneer Press Publishing Company) was an ideal setting for a retreat. The main manor was an attractive, rambling one-and-one-half-floor structure. It had seventeen spacious rooms including large living and dining rooms, a library, a sun-porch, and numerous bedrooms, some of which were master size. There were two cottages, one equipped with indoor recreational facilities and the other overlooking South Center Lake.

The manor became the center of the retreat and recovery, which allowed the guests to help one another by sharing their stories and reflecting on the Twelve Steps. At that time, the grounds consisted of 217 acres of rolling land, some of which were being cultivated and some of which remained woodland, with about a mile of lakeshore on South Center Lake. (The excellent environment bore a clear resemblance to Upland Farms.)

Lynn Carroll, a lawyer by profession, was asked to accept the position of director of Hazelden, which opened in May 1949. Personal suffering had played a significant role in his life. An alcoholic, helpless, and in despair, he emerged from the psychiatric ward of General Hospital in Minneapolis and sought the fellowship of AA at 2218, where he began his lifelong commitment to helping other alcoholics. Moving from personal calamity to a life of outstanding service to others, he became a great example of one who had a spiritual awakening and sought to carry this message to other alcoholics and to practice these principles in all his affairs.

He accepted the directorship, at great sacrifice to himself, and for three years he was the only full-time counselor. He practically lived at Hazelden, receiving occasional relief when some AA person would substitute for him. His schedule was exhausting, and the additional fund-raising efforts were frustrating. But he persevered and managed to hold things together during the critical transition from the banker Richard Lilly's hands to the purchase of Hazelden by the Butler family and the total involvement of Patrick Butler.

Carroll knew the alcoholics' needs, and he knew both experientially and cognitively the AA program. Eventually, his convictions and attitudes would conflict with what he considered the professional approach and mentality in the future development of the simple program that he had introduced. That simple program consisted of his consecutive lectures on the Twelve Steps of AA and related topics and the group discussions. Members of AA would drive up from the Twin Cities to share their own experiences of hope. It wasn't treatment; it was a retreat for the alcoholic, an opportunity to get away and reflect on what it had been like before and what was happening as they spent time engaging with one another.

Initially, Carroll's staff consisted of three people. Ann Schnable, "Ma" as she was affectionately known by the guests, helped with the cooking for the open house, but then she stayed ten years. Besides being the cook, she was a registered nurse who would dispense whatever medications were necessary and the staff psychologist who would dispense compassion, love, and discipline (no one was allowed to intrude into her kitchen). There was also a maintenance man who had been the groundskeeper for the Power family and elected to stay on. The final person was the utility man who accomplished a variety of tasks, including lifting men back into bed especially during times of withdrawal. (The original staff at The Retreat at Upland Farms consisted of five people with similar tasks.)

There was no medical staff, only a physician in St. Croix Falls they would call in case of illness. There were no attendants keeping tabs on the men; they were entitled to their personal privacy. There was only one restriction—no alcohol. Occasionally a guest would get bored, row across the lake, stop at the bar, and then, by hitching a ride, continue on his merry way to the Twin Cities.

In the early months of the new venture, Carroll grappled with the central issue that differentiates mutual help from treatment: "Should he not have some psychological or psychiatric background," either he himself or provided by some consulting professional. "There were a lot of problems I hadn't learned to work out quite right. And then I got to thinking—what the dickens! I had psychiatrists and psychologists and they didn't do me any good and I didn't know any other alcoholics that they ever did anything for" (McElrath, 1987, 31). He concluded that because he was getting good results, he would continue doing what he knew and did best. He developed a recovery course, similar to Pioneer House and 2218, based on the straight AA program and process. He would speak to the patients about the steps. It was a place where the patients would be immersed in AA.

He would talk with a patient, find out about him,

and record his impressions on a 3"×5" index card. He was able to determine who was going to stay sober and who wasn't by their attitudes. No need for voluminous intakes and multiple assessments. Carroll's patients came voluntarily, and as at Pioneer House, they were expected to stay three weeks and be immersed in AA and the Twelve Steps. (Some patients stayed just overnight but returned multiple times.) According to Carroll, the three weeks was hardly enough time to "correct some of their character defects—anger, fear, hatred, self-pity—which are the curse of the human race, not only of the alcoholic."

It was tough going for Carroll in the first years. The first Christmas after the opening, there was only one patient. Finances were a huge problem. One time driving back from the Twin Cities, he pulled over to the side of the road and practiced the third step, praying that if it be God's will, then this venture would continue.

It was Carroll's conviction that the only manner in which an alcoholic could really be helped was through the steps of AA and another alcoholic. Carroll would have a difficult time when a nonrecovering psychologist wanted to add the psychological profile of a patient— the Minnesota Multiphasic Personality Inventory (MMPI) to the treatment process and a scientific and complete medical record. As these novelties emerged, they became symbolic of the clashes between mutual help and professional treatment. Carroll looked upon these developments as the beginning of the insidious intrusion of psychological principles into the mutual help of AA and total immersion in its steps and process. Soon the Hazelden Retreat Program (the original Guest House program) would turn into the Hazelden Treatment Program.

Hazelden in its beginnings bequeathed to what would emerge as the Minnesota model: (1) the grace of a beautiful environment that promoted respect, understanding, and acceptance of the dignity of each patient; (2) a program based upon the Twelve Steps of AA; (3) the belief that time away and association with other alcoholics was central to recovery; and (4) a very simple program whose expectations were make your bed, comport yourself as a gentleman, attend the lectures on the Twelve Steps, and talk with one another about the steps and related topics. The Retreat captured much of this original simplicity.

Willmar State Hospital

While Hazelden was laying the foundation for a successful retreat of mutual help, another institution was emerging that would eventually merge with Hazelden to provide a unique breakthrough in how the United States viewed alcoholics and how they could get well.

Willmar State Hospital, established in 1912, was nestled in the rural community of Willmar in southwestern Minnesota about one hundred miles west of Minneapolis. By its original charter, one of the hospital's specific goals was the care and treatment of chronic alcoholics. As a result, Willmar State Hospital was the first of the seven state hospitals in Minnesota to serve as an inebriate asylum, the unenviable reference of that time to a treatment setting for alcoholism.

Although the hospital had been admitting alcoholics for years prior to 1950, there was no established program for alcoholics and no interest in developing one. Moreover, because it was also designated as a state hospital for mental patients, it underscored the identification of alcoholism as a mental or psychiatric problem. Before the 1950s, care at the hospital had been simply a question of holding patients, not an issue of treatment or care. This approach closely matched a similar attitude throughout the United States. The prevailing mood after the repeal of Prohibition in 1932 was one of skepticism and pessimism about alcoholics doing anything for themselves, and about doing anything for them. They needed to be institutionalized and locked in the wards with the mental patients. A more humane and caring approach within state hospitals began in Minnesota and soon became a national movement.

Shortly after Hazelden got its start, Dan Anderson, a graduate of St. Thomas College in St. Paul, was accompanying Dr. Nelson Bradley to Willmar, where the latter had been appointed superintendent in 1950. Bradley asked Anderson if he knew anything about inebriates. Anderson said no, but like any good graduate of college he said that he would look it up in the textbooks. In reality, their first decade at Willmar allowed them to create their own textbook. In the next years, the two men—Anderson, who earned his PhD in psychology, and Bradley, a psychiatrist—formed definite and progressive ideas about the treatment of alcoholics.

Both Bradley and Anderson suspected that AA could provide the answer to the recovery. Although the two men did not understand AA very well, neither its philosophy nor its comic relief and jokes, they intuitively recognized that AA's sense of humor was interwoven with deep spiritual insights. It was in this context that in the early 1950s, Bradley energetically cultivated the AA community in Willmar, the Twin Cities, and as a matter of record throughout Minnesota. Through contact with AA members, Saturday night AA meetings were organized at Willmar and speakers were recruited from AA groups statewide: Otto Zapp from St. Cloud, Pat Cronin from Pioneer House, Lynn Carroll from Hazelden, Fred Eiden from Hastings State Hospital, Pat Butler from St. Paul, whose family had been invested in Hazelden almost from the beginning, among others. The Midway Squad in St. Paul through Mel Brandes was particularly supportive of the Willmar experience. Not only did Bradley ask these men to speak, but he also asked them for their advice as he instituted the program at the hospital.

Starting in the fall of 1951, on Bradley's initiative, Willmar State Hospital sponsored a series of annual workshops to bring together professionals (doctors, nurses, clergy, and social workers) and AA people. By 1952, AA members were being encouraged to come to the hospital when the workday ended to give lectures and visit with the patients.

Bradley and Anderson were gathering the empirical evidence that AA could sober up alcoholics and sustain them in their recoveries. In AA, alcoholics were willing to tell their stories, past and present, to other alcoholics and were motivated by the practice of the twelfth step to work with other alcoholics who were still drinking. Prior to 1950, professionals had little or no success in dealing with inebriates. They simply did not know what to do with them. Bradley and Anderson saw that AA people had phenomenal insights into the thinking and personalities of alcoholics. Although the inner workings of AA had been a mystery to them, it was evident that this mutual help worked. Indeed, AA was successful in keeping many alcoholics sober.

Bradley initiated and implemented a radical departure from the psychiatric tradition in the conventional understanding of alcoholism. In rapid succession, the alcoholics were separated from the mentally ill, their doors were unlocked, and AA members were allowed to talk to the patients. Bradley and Anderson then prevailed upon the Minnesota legislature in 1954 to create paid positions called "counselors on alcoholism" whose principal credentials were their own recoveries. Minnesota was the first state to create such positions.

An Early Multidisciplinary Team

Willmar already had its physicians, nurses, psychiatrists, social workers, recreation directors, and chaplains. Now in 1954, the hospital had non-degreed counselors on alcoholism who were lay people, recovering alcoholics, having responsibility for mutual help groups, sharing responsibility for a treatment program, and having an equal say with the professional staff. This was a radical change—going from a physician-orientated, psychoanalytic hospital to a treatment program conducted by "drunks."

Another treatment strategy that gradually emerged at Willmar was the peer group: patients helped each other by simply meeting informally in small, leaderless groups. This mutual assistance and support of other patients facing similar problems could benefit any group member—one alcoholic talking to another over a cup of coffee was one of the key ingredients of mutual help at Willmar.

The new alcoholism counselors lectured on the Twelve Steps, the symptoms of alcoholism, the characteristics of alcoholic behavior, and the techniques for positive change. These gradually evolved into a formal lecture series shared by the counselors and the other members of the staff. The importance of the lectures became evident when they moved from 4:30 p.m., the end of the work day, to prime time, at 8:30 a.m.

Obviously, this team concept and activity did not take place in a day, a month, or a year. Most of the professional staff struggled with the concept of an illness, and, of course, each discipline had its professional pride and tradition of working independently. It was difficult to accept the recovering counselors as equals. By the end of the decade, however, alcoholics were recovering at Willmar and a very simple program was in place consisting of lectures, groups, individual counseling sessions, and an aftercare program in the Twin Cities.

It was an exciting period, full of exhilarating events, creative ideas, and wonderful relationships. But it was challenging. The staff was in crisis a great deal of the time, and they led a scrambling sort of existence. The people involved were never quite sure what they were doing or where they were going. Many essential parts of the Minnesota model developed quite by accident. The planning strategy was situational, individuals scurrying from one task or meeting to the next. But marvelous things were happening.

Willmar's Legacy

Willmar's legacy to the Minnesota model was (1) the idea and the potential for a multidisciplinary team, (2) a more systematic approach to the treatment of the illness, (3) the need for and value of an after-care program, and (4) the definition of alcoholism as a primary chronic illness distinct from mental illness. Essentially, Willmar's unfolding professional treatment model would slowly but surely form a symbiotic relationship with the Hazelden mutual help model, but only after some time during which it led to changes that were painful for those engaged in its evolution.

Looking back on the early days at Willmar, Bradley reflected on the esprit de corps that had been created: "I don't think our motives were any grand ones, but we had an enormous amount of support for what each other was doing. It was always the same people who stuck together—all the people who came and went over a ten-year period." For Bradley, the decade at Willmar was an adventure and what he learned he took with him and implemented in Chicago at the General Lutheran Hospital in 1960. A year later, Dan Anderson would plant the seeds for a new program at Hazelden. Four decades after that, John Curtiss opened the doors of The Retreat.

The Marriage Between Hazelden and Willmar

Pat Butler, with whom John Curtiss, as director of Fellowship Club, became quite close, was the connection between Willmar and Hazelden. He acquired Hazelden after paying off the note that the St. Paul banker, Richard Lilly, held on the Hazelden property. Butler had been visiting Willmar on a regular basis, often having Bradley and Anderson, in turn, visit with him at his home on Summit Avenue. There, they would reflect on the marvelous and strange things that were happening at their respective places. Hopeless alcoholics were getting well.

Butler forged the treatment links between Willmar State Hospital and Hazelden. He made Hazelden the beneficiary of the hospital's growing expertise. He was very aware of Bradley's innovative style as well as Bradley's uncertainty as to where everything was leading. A keen observer of people, he soon intuited the potential of the young Dan Anderson who, he believed, could both plant and cultivate new seeds from the experience that he had already garnered from Willmar. There, he had become a member of the new, but still seminal, multidisciplinary team at the State Hospital under Bradley. Butler's mission was: "To help as many alcoholics as possible, with the best care possible at the least cost possible." This was practically identical to the mission that The Retreat would later adopt.

Starting with his own recovery in 1950, Butler dedicated his life to helping as many alcoholics as he could. Most visible was his sponsorship during the 1950s of the Fellowship Club, the halfway house for men, and Dia Linn, an alcohol treatment program for women. In those early years, he was also responsible for establishing and maintaining a close relationship between Hazelden and the Yale Summer School of Alcohol Studies, despite Lynn Carroll's abiding distrust of Yale's intellectual and scientific efforts to help alcoholics.

In 1958, Butler was able to lure Anderson to the Dia Linn campus every other weekend to lecture and provide psychological testing for the women. Soon after, Anderson was visiting the Center City campus for the same reason. Then, in 1961, Butler hired Anderson as vice president and executive director of the Hazelden Foundation. In the meantime, Bradley took his experience and some of his co-workers to Chicago and launched the model at Lutheran General Hospital, which became a strong advocate and force for the multi-disciplinary approach to the treatment of the disease of alcoholism.

Anderson had to find his way. He had encountered other professional psychologists who either considered the alcoholic a lost cause or believed that alcoholism was merely a symptom of some other personality disorder. Reflecting upon those early days, Anderson recalled:

"All I know is in the early days of alcohol treatment, I was considered an inferior professional person working with alcoholics and was looked down upon." (Dr. Mann experienced similar feelings and negative remarks from his colleagues at St. Mary's.) Besides being patronized by psychologists, Anderson had to deal with the suspicions of recovering alcoholics. Among all of the professionals, the psychologist was the most threatening to the counseling staff both at Willmar and later at Hazelden in the person of Lynn Carroll and his staff.

Mutual Help and Professional Treatment

At first, the AA program was as mysterious to Dan Anderson as it was to most professionals. But Anderson was inquisitive and genuinely open. His developing insights led to his personal conviction about the value and validity of AA. He developed the ability to bridge the gap between recovering people and the professionals, unfortunately not with Lynn Carroll and his close staff. Despite the strong animosity to what he was doing, Anderson was able to bring the best methods of Willmar to the Hazelden environment.

It may be over simplistic to draw the lines between mutual help and professional treatment in the persons of Carroll and Anderson. Carroll felt everything

Anderson was introducing was an encroachment upon the mutual-help program that he had introduced and simply a multiplication of services that in no way dealt with the disease but simply psychologized it.

When Anderson came on board in 1961, he set up his office at the Fellowship Club (the Halfway House established by Pat Butler in 1953) to give Carroll the freedom to run Center City. Anderson spent his time at Dia Linn (Hazelden's treatment center for women in White Bear Lake, Minnesota, established in 1957), where he began to introduce his own ideas of treatment with a prominent role for the psychologist and the counselor. With the construction of the buildings between 1964 and 1966, Anderson began to make his presence felt at Center City, where he would prepare the staff for the treatment ideas that he wanted introduced into the new units. Carroll attended the initial meetings but over the months attended less frequently and finally withdrew completely. What upset Carroll so much was summed up by his assistant: it was the "encroachment of the down-town [Anderson's] office on the running of Hazelden." While Anderson resided at Fellowship Club, Carroll felt that his mutual-help program at Hazelden was secure.

Carroll wanted a simple and unstructured AA approach to treatment. He had no patient files, because, for him, files were a nuisance. His simple approach worked, and patients got well. But in 1966 Anderson would transplant the Willmar program, newly modified and newly adapted from Dia Linn to Center City. Lynn Carroll would have to accept it or leave. He chose the latter.

After more than fifteen years of operation under Carroll, Hazelden had a mutual help program based on AA set in a dignified, warm, human, and personally enriching environment. Dan Anderson was welding that program with his own tradition, also based substantially on AA but a treatment program systematically and structurally delivered through a multidisciplinary method.

The Professional Treatment Model

During that first decade (1966–1975) that Dan Anderson spent at Hazelden after Lynn Carroll departed, he and his associates formalized the model as represented by Hazelden. Anderson hired many of his co-workers from Willmar to create a real multidisciplinary team—nurses, chaplains, psychologists, and social workers—to blend with the recovering staff already present at little Center City where Hazelden was located.

The new buildings, which had just been finished before the beginning of this important decade, had been designed to create a therapeutic environment—similar to the Old Lodge, which generated a real sense of community and fellowship. This architectural design initiated the patient into a small mutual-help community and became a gentle daily reminder that community together with the Twelve Steps, the kit of spiritual tools, were the essentials of the recovery protocol.

Over the course of that decade, a formal treatment methodology was introduced. By 1977, Hazelden had produced a rehabilitation program that included diagnostic tools, detoxification protocols, routine medical care, psychological evaluation, individual and group counseling, family and spiritual counseling, a lecture schedule, training programs for counselors, nurses and clergy, observer programs, and marital communications workshops. Treatment gradually overshadowed the simplicity of the mutual help approach that underscored and described the early days of Hazelden under Lynn Carroll, and before him by Pat Cronin at Pioneer House. And the treatment methodology had been extended to all mood-altering chemicals, not only alcohol, thus the origin of the term *chemical dependency.*

This was the decade that laid the foundation for Hazelden's unique approach to treatment. It was one of the most exciting in all of Hazelden's history. It was a time of amazing vitality and creativity that spent itself over the entire decade and was marked by a relentless flow of new ideas and endless experimentation. It was the time also when this new Hazelden model became the most highly regarded brand of treatment in the United States with some international overtones. All of it, of course, was directed toward recovery for the alcoholic and was guided by a group of dedicated, strong-willed individuals all of whom influenced John Curtiss's recovery in one way or another and molded Hazelden's tradition, character, and personality for years to come.

Still, initially, the nonprofessional recovering counselor played the central role in therapy through personal involvement, communication, and confrontation with patients. They directed the patients toward practical ways of being honest with themselves and others. Coordinating the resources of the professional staff, the recovering counselor's role in treatment continued to be one of the distinguishing features of a treatment program based on the Minnesota model. The counselors who headed the four units as well as the Old Lodge were selected based on two criteria: (1) they had a solid recovery program and (2) they had good public speaking skills. Other professionals—chaplains, psychologists, and nurses—were hired to fill out the multidisciplinary team, which had Willmar as its model.

In the beginning, however, these counselors were often intimidated by the psychologists who read the MMPI tests every Monday morning at the meeting of the whole staff. The counselors would listen, looking uncomfortable and casting bewildered glances at one another. It seemed that the MMPI was to be the barometer of change in those early days of the multidisciplinary development and the psychologist was the program's watchdog. But the counselor had a tendency to be paranoid. (Initially the role of the psychologist was minimal. The psychologists were hired part time and worked more than one unit.) But that too passed and the lay counselor's role remained preeminent.

Just as John Curtiss was coming on board in 1979, Hazelden was becoming nationally and internationally famous and others were looking to replicate its programs. As Pat Butler remarked, the treatment center that was fashioned without a model had itself become a model for other centers around the world. The years between 1966 and 1975 were a decade of creative genius. There was little or no long-range planning as programs and buildings seemed magically to fall into place. It would be difficult to find another decade that could match up against it. It seemed that the program itself had evolved toward a synthesis of the best elements of treatment combined with the mutual help of the fellowship and the Twelve Steps of AA. Patients were treated with dignity and respect—something alcoholics could not have expected during the years when Bill W. and Dr. Bob were formulating their ideas.

This was the Hazelden that Curtiss became a part of. There were indications that the freedom to expand and create that Hazelden had experienced during this formative decade would shortly begin to suffer some constraints in the forms of licensure and accreditation. They affected not only Hazelden but also every other treatment center in the United States, including the newly established and growing treatment program established at St. Mary's hospital by Dr. George Mann.

The events of the 1980s affected Dr. Mann and Curtiss in much the same fashion. The demands of managed care and the insurance companies they represented were slowly squeezing the life out of the Minnesota treatment model. Likewise, the multiplication of services was obscuring the primary purpose for which this model was created. And the prominent roles that psychiatrists and psychologists were playing were blurring the distinctions between primary and secondary illnesses and over-pathologizing the chemically dependent person. At the same time that all of this was going on, The Retreat was seizing the future by returning to the mutual help model created by AA.

12

Acknowledgments

Current Directors

George Mann, MD, Chairman in Memorium

Terry Troy, Chairman

John Curtiss, President

Peter Vogt, MD, Vice Chairman

Robert Harvey, Secretary

Gale Sharpe, Treasurer

Robert Bisanz, Life Member

John Beal

John Brown Jr.

Fran Coyne

Judy Halabrin

Kevin Hart

Larry Hendrickson

Larry Koll

Marie Manthey

Dirk Miller, PhD

Patrick O'Neill

Joanne Sitt

Bud Premer, MD, Emeritus

Past Directors

Win Adams

Greg Amer, MD

Wally Arnetzen

Nancy Anderson

Peter Bell

Leonard Boche

George Bloom

Gretchen Bonham

Jim Clayton

Katie Collins

Michael Cowley

Jay Ecklund

Tim Forsythe

Melanie Gainsley

Richard Grey

Reverend Phil Hansen

Kathrine Hill

Keith Johnson

Dick Langlais

Patricia Levy

Ralph Neiditch

Marlene Qualle

Bill Rasmussen

Chuck Rice

Jan Schwarz

Arthur Stern

Jim Stuebner

Charlie Sweatt

Tom Van Herke

Molly Varley

Current Staff

John Curtiss, President/CEO

Diane Poole, Program Director

Debbie Johnson, Director of Operations & Finance

Patrick Dewane, Director of Development

Tara Tobin, Director of Marketing & Outreach/
Alumni Relations

Ellie Hyatt, Director of Family & Spiritual
Recovery

Mike Jamison, Director of Non-Residential Services

Sol Ryan, Director of Online Services

Jack Odom, Men's Program Coordinator

Andrea Bruner, Women's Program Coordinator

Sherry Gaugler-Stewart, Family & Spiritual Recovery Coordinator

Pamela Broz, Non-Residential Program Coordinator

Eva Monroe, Admissions Coordinator/ Supervisor–Men

Lisa Maddalena, Admissions Coordinator/ Supervisor–Women

Russell Holm, Intake & Outreach Coordinator

Jim Mendesh, Facilities Manager

Ken Chipongian, Chef Manager

Jake Klisivitch, Overnight Assistant/Security

John MacDougall, Director of Spititual Development

Stephen Crane, Older Adults Coordinator

Nan Vest, Outreach Manager–Older Adults

Dick Rice, Director of Spiritual Development (retired)

Duane (DJ) Jackson, Spiritual Director (retired)

Peter Farley, Facilities Manager (retired)

Works Cited

The primary sources for this book were the minutes of the Community of Recovering People (CORP) board meetings from 1991 to 2012.

We also want to acknowledge our debt to two scholars whose outstanding works on the history of the Alcoholics Anonymous movement are well known: Ernest Kurtz and William White and their collaborative essay, "Twelve Defining Moments in the History of Alcoholics Anonymous," published in 2008 in volume 18 of *Recent Developments in Alcoholism.*

Twelve Steps and Twelve Traditions. New York: Alcoholics Anonymous World Services, Inc. (1952).

Dr. Bob and the Good Old Timers. New York: Alcoholics Anonymous World Services, Inc. (1980).

Alcoholics Anonymous: The Big Book. New York: Alcoholics Anonymous World Services, Inc. (2002).

Bloom, S. *Creating Sanctuary: Toward the Evolution of Sane Societies.* New York: Routledge (1997).

Forrest, R. *Courage to Change.* Minneapolis: Richeson (1978).

Kurtz, E. *Not God: The History of Alcoholics Anonymous.* Center City, MN: Hazelden (1979).

McElrath, D. *Hazelden: A Spiritual Odyssey.* Center City, MN: Hazelden (1987).

_____. *Further Reflections on Hazelden's Spiritual Odyssey.* Center City, MN: Hazelden (1999).

Nakken, C. *The Addictive Personality,* 2nd ed. Center City, MN: Hazelden (1996).

White, W. L. *Slaying the Dragon: The History of Addiction Treatment and Recovery in America.* Bloomington, IL: Chestnut Health Systems Publication (1998).

About the Authors

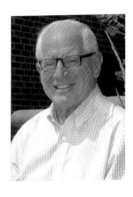

Damian McElrath, DHE

Damian McElrath spent three decades as a Franciscan priest serving the spiritual needs of others in a variety of roles, including teaching, counseling, and administrative positions. He was the president of St. Bonaventure University from 1972 to 1976. In that life, he wrote and edited a number of scholarly books and articles on historical and theological topics.

Damian arrived at Hazelden in 1977 to participate in its Clinical Pastoral Education program. Over the course of the next two decades, he served in a variety of administrative roles, including executive vice president of Recovery Services, as well as being chaplain to Hazelden's long-term program for almost a decade. He has authored a number of books on Hazelden's history, including *Hazelden: A Spiritual Odyssey*, as well as biographies of its founders, Patrick Butler and Dan Anderson. Damian authored and edited *The Story Behind the Little Black Book* as well as *The Story Behind the Little Red Book*. His most recent book, *The Essence of Twelve Step Recovery*, is about the spiritual foundation of the Twelve Step Program.

Damian has served as a spiritual coordinator at The Retreat since 2011, hearing Fifth Steps and providing spiritual guidance to the guests.

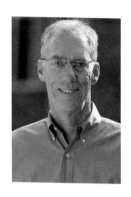

John H. Curtiss, MA, LADC

John is president of the Community of Recovering People board of directors and of The Retreat. He has been a member of the CORP board since its beginnings, and is one of the principle designers of The Retreat model of care. Prior to beginning his employment with CORP in April 1998, John was employed by the Hazelden Foundation for over nineteen years. In his years at Hazelden, John served in a variety of roles, including: vice president of Hazelden's National Continuum, executive director of Hazelden's Outreach Services, executive director of Fellowship Club, Hazelden's intermediate care facility in St. Paul, unit supervisor of two of Hazelden's primary treatment units and as a chemical dependency counselor. John was also an instructor in Hazelden's professional education program, teaching group therapy, advanced counseling skills, and the treatment of special populations.

John has a masters degree in human and health services administration from Saint Mary's University of Minnesota; he's a graduate of Hazelden's Counselor Training Program. He is a licensed counselor in the state of Minnesota and is a nationally certified recovery specialist.

John has served on numerous boards, including Community of Recovering People and Sobriety High School; he is the past president of the Association of Halfway House Alcohol Programs of North America (AHHAP) and current chair of the Minnesota Association of Sober Homes (MASH). He has served as guest faculty for Rutgers Summer School for Advanced Addiction Studies and is the co-author of a Hazelden publication titled "Letting Go."

John has dedicated his life to the creation of affordable, accessible recovery communities throughout the United States and many other countries. He led the efforts to set up Hazelden's treatment continuum in New York City and Chicago and their intermediate care program in West Palm Beach, Florida.

The Retreat model of recovery is rapidly becoming a national standard for a non-clinical, spiritually grounded, affordable approach to helping people access recovery from alcohol and drug dependency. The Retreat has captured the hearts of recovering alcoholics and professionals throughout the country. It has gained a reputation, not only as an affordable, effective approach to helping people recover, but as a great place for alcoholics in recovery to be of service to others.

John has consulted with many individuals and organizations throughout the United States and abroad interested in replicating The Retreat model of recovery. Programs modeling themselves after The Retreat model now exist in Hong Kong; New Zealand; Sioux Falls, South Dakota; Vero Beach, Florida; and Nashville, with upcoming projects in Dallas and Sydney.